MASTERING NURSING MEDICAL - SURGICAL
PROCEDURES
(From Classroom to Patient Care Excellence)

A COMPREHENSIVE GUIDE FOR BACHELOR'S AND MASTER'S STUDENTS

Dr. Joshua G. Kaya
Dr Brandi J. Gresham

Copyright ©

All rights reserved. This work, including but not limited to text, graphics, and images, is the intellectual property of Dr. Joshua G. Kaya and Dr. Brandi J. Gresham. It is protected by copyright laws and international treaties. Unauthorized reproduction, distribution, or modification of this work, in whole or in part, is strictly prohibited and may result in civil and criminal penalties. Copyright © 2024 by Dr. Joshua G. Kaya and Dr. Brandi J. Gresham.

Preface

In medical-surgical nursing. Dr. Joshua G. Kaya and Dr. Brandi J. Gresham, the co-authors of this work, have dedicated their careers to advancing nursing education and practice.

This text is designed to be a companion for students embarking on their journey in nursing, whether pursuing a Bachelor's or Master's degree. It serves as a roadmap, guiding students through the intricacies of medical-surgical procedures with clarity and depth. Each chapter is meticulously crafted to offer a blend of theoretical insights, evidence-based practices, and practical application.

We recognize that the field of nursing is dynamic, with new research and technologies constantly shaping clinical practice. Therefore, this guide is not meant to be static but rather a living document that evolves with the changing landscape of healthcare. It is our hope that students will use this book as a springboard for further exploration and innovation in the field.

Throughout these pages, we emphasize the importance of critical thinking, clinical reasoning, and holistic patient care. Nursing is not just about mastering procedures; it's about understanding the underlying principles and implications for patient outcomes. As such, we encourage students to approach each topic with curiosity, empathy, and a commitment to lifelong learning.

We would like to express our gratitude to the students and colleagues who have inspired and challenged us along the way. Your dedication to the nursing profession fuels our passion for education and drives us to continually strive for excellence.

In closing, we invite students to embark on this educational journey with an open mind and a willingness to engage deeply with the material. By mastering the principles and practices outlined in this guide, we believe that you will be well-equipped to meet the challenges and opportunities that lie ahead in your nursing career.

Sincerely,

Dr. Joshua G. Kaya
Dr. Brandi J. Gresham

EDITORIAL OVERVIEW

Dear colleagues and esteemed students pursuing degrees in Medical Nursing at both undergraduate and master's levels, It is with great pleasure and enthusiasm that I introduce myself as the editor of our forthcoming textbook on medical-surgical procedures for nursing students. My name is Dr. Jackie A. Larson, and I am honored to serve as the editor of this comprehensive guide aimed at enhancing the education and clinical practice of nursing students in both Bachelor's and Master's programs.

With years of experience in the field of medicine, particularly in surgical care and medical education, I bring a wealth of knowledge and expertise to this project. Throughout my career, I have been dedicated to advancing medical knowledge and improving patient outcomes through education, research, and clinical practice. As an educator and practitioner, I understand the importance of providing nursing students with a solid foundation in medical-surgical procedures, equipping them with the skills and confidence needed to deliver high-quality patient care.

This textbook represents a collaborative effort among experts in the field, each contributing their unique insights and experiences to create a comprehensive resource that covers a wide range of topics relevant to medical-surgical nursing. From fundamental principles to advanced techniques, our aim is to provide students with a thorough understanding of medical-surgical procedures, preparing them to excel in their future careers as healthcare professionals.

I am grateful for the opportunity to work with such a talented team of authors, whose dedication and expertise have been instrumental in bringing this project to fruition. Together, we have meticulously crafted a textbook that is both informative and engaging, incorporating the latest evidence-based practices and clinical guidelines to ensure its relevance and applicability in today's healthcare environment.

I am confident that this textbook will serve as an invaluable resource for nursing students at all levels of their education, offering a comprehensive overview of medical-surgical procedures and empowering them to deliver safe, effective, and compassionate care to their patients.

Thank you for your support and collaboration throughout this process. I look forward to the continued success of this project and the positive impact it will have on the education and training of future generations of nursing professionals.

Sincerely,

Dr. Jackie A. Larson

Table of Contents

Preface
  - Editorial Overview

Acquired Immunodeficiency Syndrome (AIDS)
  - Introduction
  - Pathophysiology
  - Classification of HIV Disease Stages
  - Risk Factors
  - Clinical Manifestations
  - Assessment and Diagnostic Methods
  - Medical Management

Antidepressant Therapy
  - Introduction
  - Types of Antidepressants
  - Considerations in Antidepressant Therapy
  - Electroconvulsive Therapy

Nutrition Therapy
- Introduction
- Nutritional Requirements for Patients with AIDS
- Dietary Modifications
- Appetite Stimulants and Oral Supplements

Nursing Process for Patients with HIV/AIDS
- Assessment
- Nutritional Status
- Skin and Mucous Membranes
- Respiratory Status
- Neurologic Status
- Fluid and Electrolyte Status
- Level of Knowledge
- Use of Alternative Therapies
- Diagnosis
- Collaborative Problems/Potential Complications
- Planning and Goals
- Nursing Interventions
- Continuing Care
- Evaluation

Medical Management of Myocardial Infarction
- Introduction
- Objectives of Medical Management
- Reperfusion Strategies
- Pharmacologic Therapy
- Invasive Procedures
- Nursing Management

Addison's Disease
- Definition and Causes
- Symptoms and Complications

Assessment and Diagnostic Findings
- Plasma ACTH Levels
- Serum Cortisol Levels
- Electrolyte Imbalances

Medical Management
- Immediate Treatment for Circulatory Shock
- Long-Term Corticosteroid Replacement

- Antibiotics for Infection

Nursing Management
- Fluid Balance Assessment
- Monitoring for Addisonian Crisis
- Patient Education on Stress Avoidance

Alzheimer's Disease: Clinical Manifestations and Diagnosis
- Progressive Neurologic Disorder
- Familial vs. Sporadic Forms
- Symptoms and Diagnostic Tools

Medical Management of Alzheimer's Disease
- Cholinesterase Inhibitors
- Nursing Interventions for Cognitive Support

Nursing Process for Alzheimer's Disease
- Comprehensive Assessment
- Nursing Diagnoses and Planning
- Interventions and Patient Education

Medical Management of Anemia
   - Packed Red Blood Cell Transfusions
   - Gerontologic Considerations

Nursing Process for Anemic Patients
   - Assessment and Diagnostic Evaluation
   - Nursing Diagnoses and Goals
   - Interventions for Fatigue Management and Nutrition

Management of Iron Deficiency Anemia
   - Causes and Clinical Manifestations
   - Diagnostic Methods and Medical Management
   - Nursing Interventions and Patient Education

Management of Megaloblastic Anemia
   - Folic Acid and Vitamin B12 Deficiency
   - Pathophysiology and Assessment
   - Medical and Nursing Management

Management of Sickle Cell Anemia

- Pathophysiology and Clinical Manifestations
- Diagnostic Findings and Medical Treatment
- Nursing Process for Sickle Cell Crisis

Assessment and Management of Arterial Embolism and Thrombosis
- Clinical Manifestations and Medical Management
- Nursing Interventions and Risk Factor Modification

Understanding Arteriosclerosis and Atherosclerosis
- Pathophysiology and Risk Factors
- Clinical Manifestations and Management Strategies

Nursing Care for Rheumatoid Arthritis
- Clinical Manifestations and Diagnostic Methods
- Medical and Nursing Management
- Home Care and Patient Education

Promoting Home- and Community-Based Care
   - Patient Education and Continuing Care
   - Referral to Home Care Services

Asthma: Overview and Epidemiology
   - Definition, Risk Factors, and Complications

Assessment, Diagnosis, and Medical Management of Asthma
   - Symptoms, Types, and Diagnostic Methods
   - Pharmacologic Therapy and Nursing Management

Home and Community Care for Asthma
   - Patient Education and Self-Care
   - Follow-Up Appointments and Support Groups

Status Asthmaticus: Emergency Management

- Immediate Interventions and Medical Treatment

- Understanding Benign Prostatic Hyperplasia (BPH) and its Impact

Clinical Manifestations of BPH
- Recognizing Symptoms: From Urinary Changes to Complications

Assessment and Diagnostic Methods
- Tools and Techniques for Diagnosing BPH

Medical Management of BPH
- Exploring Treatment Options: From Conservative to Surgical Approaches

Nursing Management of BPH
- Nursing Strategies for Supporting Patients with BPH

Prostatectomy
- Overview of Prostatectomy: Indications and Considerations

Types of Prostatectomy
- Exploring Surgical Approaches
Preoperative Preparation
- Getting Ready for Surgery: Assessments, Education, and Planning

Intraoperative Care
- Supporting Patients During Surgery: Nursing Roles and Responsibilities

Postoperative Care
- Recovery and Beyond: Nursing Interventions for Prostatectomy Patients

Complications and Follow-up
- Managing Complications and Ensuring Continued Care

Buerger's Disease (Thromboangiitis Obliterans)

- Understanding the Characteristics and Demographics

Clinical Manifestations of Buerger's Disease
- Recognizing the Symptoms: From Pain to Ulceration

Assessment and Diagnosis
- Diagnostic Methods: Tools and Techniques for Identifying Buerger's Disease

Medical Management of Buerger's Disease
- Objectives and Interventions for Improving Circulation and Extremity Protection

Nursing Management of Buerger's Disease
- Supportive Care and Preventive Measures for Patients with Buerger's Disease

Assessing Patient and Family Understanding and Coping
- Strategies for Assessing and Supporting Patients and Families

Monitoring and Managing Potential Complications

- Proactive Approaches to Complication Detection and Management

Nursing Management: Acute Phase
- Priorities and Interventions During the Acute Phase of Buerger's Disease

Nursing Process: Rehabilitation Phase
- Comprehensive Care Strategies for the Rehabilitation Phase

Promoting Nutrition
- Teaching and Strategies for Improving Nutrition in Buerger's Disease Patients

Relieving Pain
- Multidisciplinary Approaches and Pain Relief Strategies

Decreasing Fatigue
- Understanding and Addressing Fatigue in Buerger's Disease Patients

Improving Body Image and Self-Esteem

- Strategies for Supporting Body Image and Self-Esteem in Buerger's Disease Patients

Assisting in Grieving
- Emotional Support and Coping Assistance for Patients and Families

Monitoring and Managing Potential Complications
- Proactive Measures for Complication Management

Promoting Home- and Community-Based Care
- Education and Support for Transitioning to Home Care

Nursing Management Related to Treatment
- Nursing Interventions for Various Treatment Modalities

Cancer of the Bladder
- Clinical Manifestations, Assessment
- Diagnostic Methods

- Medical and Nursing Management

Cancer of the Breast
- Risk Factors
- Prevention Strategies
- Clinical Manifestations
- Assessment
- Diagnostic Methods
- Medical and Nursing Management

Nursing Process: The Patient Undergoing Surgery for Breast Cancer
- Assessment
- Diagnosis
- Planning and Goals
- Preoperative and Postoperative - Nursing Interventions, Home and Community-Based Care
- Evaluation

Colorectal Cancer
- Clinical Manifestations
- Assessment and Diagnostic Methods

- Gerontologic Considerations
- Medical Management
- Surgical Management
- Nursing Process: The Patient Undergoing Hysterectomy
- Nursing Process: The Patient with Colorectal Cancer

Prostate Cancer
- Overview
- Medical Management
- Nursing Process for Patient Undergoing Prostatectomy
- Patient Education and Home Care

Malignant Melanoma
- Assessment
- Diagnosis
- Planning and Goals
- Nursing Interventions
- Evaluation

Stomach Cancer
- Assessment

- Diagnosis
- Planning and Goals
- Nursing Interventions
- Promoting Home- and Community-Based Care

Testicular Cancer
- Clinical Manifestations
- Assessment and Diagnostic Methods
- Medical Management
- Nursing Management

Nursing Process: The Patient with a Cardiac Myopathy
- Assessment
- Diagnosis
- Planning and Goals
- Nursing Interventions
- Promoting Home- and Community-Based Care

Cancer Surgery (General)
- Overview
- Nursing Process:

- Assessment
-Diagnosis Planning,
- Interventions, Evaluation

Cataract
- Overview
- Medical and Surgical Management

Cerebrovascular Accident (CVA)
- Overview
- Medical Management

Nursing Process: The Patient Recovering from an Ischemic Stroke

Cholelithiasis and Cholecystitis
- Overview
- Assessment and Diagnosis
- Medical Management

Nursing Process for Guillain-Barré Syndrome (GBS)

Assessment

- Nursing Diagnoses

Collaborative Problems/Potential Complications:

- Respiratory compromise requiring mechanical ventilation.
- Autonomic dysfunction leading to dysrhythmias or hypotension.
- Thrombosis due to immobility.

Planning and Goals:

Nursing Interventions:

- Preventing Aspiration:
    - Minimizing Injury Risk:
    - Addressing Anxiety:

Evaluation:

nursing Process: The Patient with Guillain-Barré Syndrome (GBS)**
- Assessment (Ongoing and Critical)
- Monitoring for Complications - Diagnosis
- Nursing Diagnoses
- Collaborative Problems/Potential Complications function
- Nursing Interventions
- Potential Complications
- Promoting Home- and Community-Based Care
- Teaching Patients Self-Care
- Evaluation
- Expected Outcomes

Nursing Process: The Patient with Traumatic Brain Injury (TBI)
- Assessment
- Diagnosis
- Nursing Diagnoses

- Nursing Interventions
- Monitoring and Managing Complications
- Promoting Home- and Community-Based Care
  - Evaluation
    - Expected Outcomes

Nursing Process: The Patient with Heart Failure
  - Assessment
  - Nursing Diagnoses
  - Collaborative Problems/Potential Complications
  - Planning and Goals
  - Nursing Interventions
  - Promoting Home- and Community-Based Care
    - Evaluation
      - Expected Outcomes

Nursing Process: The Patient with an Esophageal Condition and Reflux
  - Assessment
  - Diagnosis: Nursing Diagnoses

- Planning and Goals
- Nursing Interventions
- Evaluation
  - Expected Patient Outcomes

Other Conditions
- Subdural Hematoma
- Intracerebral Hemorrhage and Hematoma
- Medical Management (ICP Management)
- Hemophilia
- Hepatic Encephalopathy
- Hiatal Hernia
- Hodgkin's Disease
- Huntington Disease
- Hyperglycemic Hyperosmolar Nonketotic Syndrome
- Hypertension

Nursing Process for Hypertension

Assessment

- Nursing Diagnoses
- Collaborative Problems/Potential Complications

Planning and Goals
- Patient understanding of disease process and treatment
- Nursing Interventions
- Evaluation

Nursing Process for Mitral Stenosis

- Clinical Manifestations
- Assessment and Diagnostic Methods
- Medical Management
- Symptom management
- Anticoagulation
- Exercise restrictions
- Surgical intervention

Nursing Management

Multiple Myeloma

- Clinical Manifestations

- Assessment and Diagnostic Methods
- Medical Management
- Nursing Management

Multiple Sclerosis (MS)
- Pathophysiology
- Disease Course
- Clinical Manifestations
- Assessment and Diagnostic Findings
- Medical Management
- Nursing Management

Nursing Process: The Patient with a Spontaneous Vertebral Fracture Related to Osteoporosis

- Assessment
- Nursing Diagnoses
- Planning and Goals
- Nursing Interventions
-

Promoting Understanding of Osteoporosis
- Relieving Pain
- Improving Bowel Elimination

- Preventing Injury
- Evaluation

Acute Otitis Media

- Clinical Manifestations
- Management

Chronic Otitis Media

- Clinical Manifestations
- Medical Management
- Nursing Management

Pancreatitis
- Clinical Manifestations
- Assessment and Diagnostic Findings
- Medical Management
- Nursing Management

Chronic Pancreatitis
- Clinical Manifestations
- Medical Management
- Nursing Management

Parkinson's Disease

- Clinical Manifestations
- Assessment and Diagnostic Methods
- Medical Management

Parkinson's Disease
- Clinical Manifestations
- Assessment and Diagnostic Methods
- Medical Management
  - Surgical interventions

Nursing Process: The Patient with Parkinson's Disease
  - Assessment
  - Nursing Diagnoses
  - Planning and Goals
  - Nursing Interventions
  - Promoting Home- and Community-Based Care
  - Evaluation

Pelvic Inflammatory Disease (PID)

- Pathophysiology
- Clinical Manifestations
- Complications
- Medical Management
- Nursing Management

Pemphigus

- Pathophysiology
- Clinical Manifestations
- Assessment and Diagnostic Findings
- Medical Management

Nursing Process: The Patient with Pemphigus

Peptic Ulcer

- Clinical Manifestations
- Assessment and Diagnostic Methods
- Medical Management

Pericarditis

Nursing Process: The Patient with Pericarditis
- Assessment
- Diagnosis
- Planning and Goals
- Nursing Interventions
- Evaluation

Preoperative Concerns

Nursing Process: The Patient with Pericarditis:

Assessment
- Pain Assessment
- Pericardial Friction Rub
- Temperature Monitoring###

- Nursing Diagnoses
- Planning and Goals
- Nursing Interventions
- Evaluation:

Pulmonary Arterial Hypertension (PAH)
Introduction
- Clinical Manifestations
- Assessment and Diagnostic Methods
- Medical Management
- Nursing Management

Acquired Immunodeficiency Syndrome (AIDS)

Introduction

AIDS represents the most severe manifestation within a spectrum of illnesses linked to human immunodeficiency virus (HIV) infection.

Pathophysiology

- HIV is a retrovirus carrying genetic material in RNA.
- Infection occurs when HIV infiltrates host CD4 (T) cells, prompting viral replication and affecting other CD4 cells.

Classification of HIV Disease Stages

- Primary infection
- HIV asymptomatic
- HIV symptomatic

- AIDS

Risk Factors

- Transmission through bodily fluids via high-risk behaviors.
- Includes heterosexual intercourse, injection drug use, male homosexual relations, blood transfusions, and healthcare worker exposures.

Clinical Manifestations

Respiratory:

- Symptoms include shortness of breath, cough, chest pain, and fever.
- Opportunistic infections like Pneumocystis jiroveci (PCP), Mycobacterium avium-intracellulare, and cytomegalovirus (CMV) are common.

Gastrointestinal:

- Manifestations include loss of appetite, nausea, vomiting, oral/esophageal candidiasis, chronic diarrhea, weight loss, and perianal skin excoriation.

Wasting Syndrome (Cachexia):

- Marked by involuntary weight loss, chronic diarrhea, or chronic weakness with fever.

Oncologic:

- Prevalent cancers include Kaposi's sarcoma, B-cell lymphomas, and invasive cervical cancer.

Neurologic:

- Neurocognitive disorders, peripheral neuropathy, HIV encephalopathy, and infections like cryptococcal meningitis and progressive multifocal leukoencephalopathy (PML) occur.

Assessment and Diagnostic Methods

- Enzyme immunoassay (EIA), Western blot assay, viral load tests, and saliva tests confirm HIV antibodies.

Medical Management

- Treatment involves HAART, antimicrobial therapy, and management of specific infections and complications.
- Chemoprophylaxis, antidiarrheal therapy, and chemotherapy may be necessary.

Conclusion

Understanding the pathophysiology, clinical manifestations, and management of AIDS is crucial for effective patient care and prevention strategies.

#Antidepressant Therapy:
Depression treatment involves psychotherapy alongside pharmacotherapy, including antidepressants like imipramine, desipramine,

fluoxetine, and possibly psychostimulants. Electroconvulsive therapy may be considered for severe, treatment-resistant depression.

#Nutrition Therapy:
A tailored, nutritious diet is crucial. Patients with diarrhea should consume low-fat, low-lactose, low-insoluble fiber, and low-caffeine diets, with calorie counts used to evaluate and manage unexplained weight loss. Appetite stimulants and oral supplements can address AIDS-related anorexia and dietary deficiencies.

Nursing Process for Patients with HIV/AIDS:

Assessment:
- Identify potential risk factors, including sexual practices and history of IV/injection drug use.
- Evaluate both physical and psychological status thoroughly.
- Investigate factors impacting the immune system functioning comprehensively.

Nutritional Status:
- Gather a detailed dietary history.
- Identify barriers to oral intake such as anorexia, nausea, vomiting, oral pain, or swallowing difficulties.
- Assess the patient's ability to access and prepare food.
- Assess nutritional status using weight, anthropometric measurements (e.g., triceps skinfold), and laboratory tests including BUN, serum protein, albumin, and transferrin levels.

Skin and Mucous Membranes:

- Perform daily inspections for breakdown, ulcers, and signs of infection.
- Monitor the oral cavity for redness, ulcerations, and candidiasis.
- Evaluate the perianal area for excoriation and infection.
- Obtain wound cultures to identify infectious organisms if necessary.

Respiratory Status:
- Monitor for respiratory symptoms such as cough, sputum production, shortness of breath, orthopnea, tachypnea, and chest pain.
- Assess pulmonary function through various means including chest x-rays, ABGs, pulse oximetry, and pulmonary function tests.

Neurologic Status:
- Assess mental status, including level of consciousness, orientation, and memory function.
- Watch for sensory deficits such as visual changes, headaches, and numbness or tingling in the extremities.

- Observe motor impairments like altered gait and weakness.
- Monitor for seizure activity.

Fluid and Electrolyte Status:
- Check skin and mucous membrane turgor and moisture levels.
- Look for signs of dehydration such as increased thirst, decreased urine output, low blood pressure, rapid weak pulse, or changes in urine specific gravity.
- Monitor electrolyte levels and assess for deficits, indicated by symptoms such as altered mental status, muscle twitching, cramps, irregular pulse, nausea, vomiting, and shallow respirations.

Level of Knowledge:
- Evaluate patient and family/friends' understanding of HIV/AIDS and its transmission.
- Assess a patient's reaction to diagnosis and coping mechanisms.
- Identify available support resources.

Use of Alternative Therapies:
- Inquire about any alternative therapies being used.
- Encourage patients to report alternative therapy use to their primary healthcare provider.
- Familiarize yourself with potential side effects and discuss with the patient and healthcare team if suspected side effects arise.
- Maintain an open-minded approach to alternative therapies and acknowledge their importance to the patient.

Diagnosis:
Nursing diagnoses for patients with HIV/AIDS encompass various aspects of physical and psychological well-being:
- Impaired skin integrity due to cutaneous manifestations of HIV infection, excoriation, and diarrhea.
- Diarrhea related to enteric pathogens or HIV infection.
- Risk for infection due to immunodeficiency.

- Activity intolerance resulting from weakness, fatigue, malnutrition, impaired fluid and electrolyte balance, and hypoxia associated with pulmonary infections.
- Disturbed thought processes linked to shortened attention span, impaired memory, confusion, and disorientation from HIV encephalopathy.
- Ineffective airway clearance due to conditions like PCP, increased bronchial secretions, and decreased ability to cough associated with weakness and fatigue.
- Pain arising from impaired perianal skin integrity secondary to diarrhea, KS, and peripheral neuropathy.
- Imbalanced nutrition, less than body requirements, due to decreased oral intake.
- Social isolation stemming from the stigma of the disease, withdrawal of support systems, isolation procedures, and fear of infecting others.
- Anticipatory grieving triggered by changes in lifestyle and roles, along with an unfavorable prognosis.

- Deficient knowledge regarding HIV infection, methods of preventing transmission, and self-care.

Collaborative Problems/Potential Complications:
Potential complications for patients with HIV/AIDS include opportunistic infections, impaired breathing or respiratory failure, wasting syndrome, fluid and electrolyte imbalances, and adverse reactions to medications.

Planning and Goals:
Goals for patients may involve achieving and maintaining skin integrity, resuming usual bowel patterns, preventing infection, improving activity tolerance, enhancing thought processes, promoting airway clearance, alleviating pain, improving nutritional status, increasing socialization, expressing grief, enhancing knowledge regarding disease prevention and self-care, and preventing complications.

Nursing Interventions:
Interventions aim to address various aspects of patient care:

- Promoting skin integrity through regular assessments, oral care, positioning, pressure-relieving devices, skincare practices, and appropriate footwear.
- Maintaining perianal skin integrity by assessing, cleansing, promoting hygiene, applying topical treatments, and monitoring for infection.
- Promoting usual bowel patterns by assessing, counseling, monitoring stool volume, recommending dietary changes, administering medications, and assessing self-care strategies.
- Preventing infection by educating patients and caregivers, monitoring for signs and symptoms, obtaining cultures, encouraging safe sexual practices, discouraging IV drug use, and maintaining aseptic technique.
- Improving activity tolerance through monitoring, planning daily routines, teaching energy conservation techniques, and reducing anxiety using relaxation methods.

Collaboration with other healthcare team members is essential to identify and address factors contributing to fatigue, such as anemia, which may be managed with interventions like epoetin alfa (Epogen).

Maintaining Thought Processes:
- Regularly assess mental status and provide reorientation as needed.
- Maintain a consistent daily schedule and provide clear, simple instructions.
- Ensure a safe environment with adequate lighting and plan engaging activities.

Improving Airway Clearance:
- Assess respiratory status, cough, and sputum characteristics daily.
- Provide pulmonary therapy every 2 hours to prevent secretion stasis and promote airway clearance.
- Position the patient in a manner conducive to breathing and airway clearance.
- Encourage adequate rest, evaluate fluid intake, and provide humidified oxygen or mechanical ventilation if necessary.

Relieving Pain and Discomfort:
- Assess pain severity and its impact on various aspects of the patient's life.
- Offer comfort measures such as soft cushions, topical anesthetics, and avoidance of irritating foods.
- Administer analgesics and nonpharmacologic interventions to manage pain effectively.

Improving Nutritional Status:
- Monitor weight, dietary intake, and laboratory values to assess nutritional status.
- Implement measures to facilitate oral intake and control nausea and vomiting.
- Encourage supplementation and provide enteral or parenteral feedings as needed.

Decreasing Social Isolation:
- Foster an atmosphere of acceptance and understanding for patients with AIDS and their families.
- Encourage patients to express their feelings and assure them that isolation is common but not unique.

- Educate patients, families, and friends about the modes of HIV transmission to reduce stigma and fear.

Coping With Grief:
- Help patients identify support resources and coping mechanisms.
- Encourage continued social interaction and engagement in usual activities.
- Suggest participation in support groups and hotlines for additional support.

Monitoring and Managing Potential Complications:
- Educate patients about signs and symptoms of opportunistic infections and the importance of prompt reporting.
- Monitor respiratory status, fluid balance, and medication side effects closely and intervene as necessary.
- Provide comprehensive information about medications and their side effects while monitoring laboratory values regularly.

Promoting Home- and Community-Based Care:
- Assist patients in transitioning to home care settings with appropriate support services and resources.

Teaching Patients Self-Care:

Educate patients, families, and friends thoroughly about HIV/AIDS, addressing fears and misconceptions, and discussing transmission prevention measures.

Discuss precautions such as condom use during sexual intercourse, avoiding oral contact with bodily fluids, and steering clear of sexual practices that may cause cuts or tears.

Provide instructions on hand hygiene and safe handling of items soiled with bodily fluids to prevent disease transmission.

Emphasize the importance of adhering to medication regimens and assisting patients and caregivers in integrating these into their daily lives.

Teach medication administration techniques, including IV preparations, and provide guidelines on infection control, follow-up care, diet, rest, and activities.

Instruct on the administration of enteral or parenteral feedings if necessary, and offer support and guidance for coping with the disease.

Continuing Care:

Refer patients and families to home care nursing or hospice services for physical and emotional support.

Assist family and caregivers in providing supportive care, including administering medications, managing nutrition, wound care, and respiratory support.

Provide emotional support to patients and families and refer them to community programs for additional assistance such as housekeeping, transportation, and therapy.

Encourage discussions about end-of-life decisions and provide resources for legal and financial assistance.

Evaluation:

Expected outcomes include maintaining skin integrity, resuming usual bowel habits, remaining free of infections, maintaining adequate activity tolerance and thought processes, effective airway clearance, decreased pain, maintaining nutritional status, decreased social isolation, progressing through grieving process, increased understanding of AIDS, and remaining free of complications.

Medical Management:

The objectives of medical management aim to minimize myocardial damage, preserve myocardial function, and prevent complications such as lethal dysrhythmias and cardiogenic shock.

Reperfusion strategies involve the emergency use of thrombolytic medications or percutaneous coronary intervention (PCI) to restore blood flow to the affected myocardial tissue.

Efforts to reduce myocardial oxygen demand and increase oxygen supply include the administration of medications such as nitrates (nitroglycerin), oxygen therapy, and bed rest.

Invasive procedures like coronary artery bypass grafting (CABG) or minimally invasive direct coronary artery bypass (MIDCAB) may be considered in certain cases.

Pharmacologic therapy includes:

- Nitrates (such as nitroglycerin) to increase oxygen supply to the myocardium.
- Anticoagulants like aspirin and heparin to prevent further clot formation.
- Analgesics, particularly morphine sulfate, to alleviate chest pain and discomfort.
- Angiotensin-converting enzyme (ACE) inhibitors to improve cardiac function and reduce myocardial workload.
- Beta-blockers, initially administered during acute management and continued post-hospital discharge, to reduce heart rate, blood pressure, and myocardial oxygen demand.

Thrombolytic agents such as alteplase (t-PA, Activase) and reteplase (r-PA, TNKase) are crucial in dissolving blood clots but must be administered promptly, ideally within 3 to 6 hours of symptom onset, to be most effective.

Nursing Management

In nursing management, it's crucial to closely monitor patients and regularly assess the effectiveness of treatments like oxygen administration and chest physiotherapy. Additionally, consider the patient's other needs such as positioning and managing anxiety. Be vigilant for any ventilation problems that could cause anxiety, and if necessary, administer sedation or, as a last resort, paralytic agents with proper sedation and pain management. Monitor patients on paralytic agents closely to prevent complications and ensure their comfort.

Addison's disease

Addison's disease results from insufficient adrenal cortex function due to various causes like autoimmune atrophy or therapeutic corticosteroid use. Symptoms include muscle weakness, GI issues, fatigue, and electrolyte imbalances. In severe cases, it can lead to an Addisonian crisis, characterized by circulatory shock, abdominal symptoms, confusion, and potential life-threatening complications triggered by stressors like surgery or dehydration.

In the assessment and diagnostic findings of Addison's Disease, indicators include elevated plasma ACTH levels, decreased serum cortisol levels, and imbalances in glucose, sodium, and potassium levels, along with leukocytosis. Immediate medical management targets circulatory shock by restoring blood circulation through fluid administration and corticosteroids, with IV hydrocortisone followed by glucose solutions. Antibiotics may be necessary if infection is a trigger. Long-term treatment involves lifelong corticosteroid and mineralocorticoid replacement. Nursing management entails assessing fluid balance and stress, monitoring for signs of crisis, and advising patients to avoid stressors. Treatment during a crisis involves fluid, glucose, electrolyte replacement, and hormone therapy. Home care includes educating patients and families on medication management, dietary adjustments, and recognizing signs of hormone imbalance. Additionally, continuing care involves follow-up assessments and health promotion activities.

Alzheimer's disease

Alzheimer's disease (AD) is a progressive neurologic disorder characterized by cognitive decline and behavioral changes. Despite being more common with age, it's not a natural part of aging. Various factors such as genetics, lifestyle, and inflammation contribute to its development. AD presents in two forms: familial, affecting less than 10% of cases, and sporadic, the more common late-onset type.

Clinical manifestations vary widely, starting with forgetfulness and progressing to communication difficulties, personality changes, and eventually reliance on others for daily tasks. Diagnosis relies on excluding other conditions and assessing symptoms through medical history, physical examination, and cognitive tests like the Mini-Mental Status Examination. Diagnostic tools include EEG, CT scans, MRIs, and laboratory tests, though definitive confirmation often requires autopsy.

Alzheimer's disease (AD) presents significant challenges in medical management due to its progressive nature and the lack of a cure. Treatment primarily focuses on managing cognitive symptoms using cholinesterase inhibitors like donepezil hydrochloride (Aricept) and memantine (Namenda). These drugs aim to enhance acetylcholine uptake in the brain to maintain memory skills for a period. Nursing interventions for patients with AD encompass various aspects of care to support cognitive function, ensure physical safety, reduce anxiety and agitation, promote independence in self-care activities, improve communication, provide socialization opportunities, ensure adequate nutrition, balance activity and rest, and offer support for home and community-based care. Evaluation of patient outcomes includes maintaining cognitive, functional, and social interaction abilities, preventing injuries, facilitating self-care participation, managing anxiety and agitation, ensuring effective communication, meeting socialization and intimacy needs, maintaining adequate nutrition, activity, and rest, and ensuring patient and family caregivers are knowledgeable about the condition and treatment regimens.

In the nursing process for patients with Alzheimer's disease (AD), thorough assessment is pivotal, involving a comprehensive health history, mental status examination, and physical assessment to detect symptoms indicative of dementia. These findings are then conveyed to the physician, and assistance with diagnostic evaluation is provided as necessary, promoting a calm environment to enhance patient safety and cooperation. Nursing diagnoses encompass a range of concerns including impaired thought processes, risk for injury, anxiety, imbalanced nutrition, activity intolerance, deficient self-care, impaired social interaction, deficient knowledge of family/caregiver, and ineffective family processes. Planning and goals revolve around supporting cognitive function, ensuring physical safety, reducing anxiety and agitation, promoting adequate nutrition and communication, enhancing self-care and socialization, and educating caregivers. Nursing interventions are diverse, aiming to support cognitive function by creating a calm and predictable environment, promoting physical safety by removing hazards and providing supervision, supporting independence in self-care activities, reducing anxiety and agitation through emotional support and environmental adjustments, improving communication by minimizing distractions, facilitating socialization and intimacy, promoting adequate nutrition, balancing activity and rest, and providing support for home- and community-based care, while being attentive to the emotional challenges faced by the family.

Medical Management of Anemia

Medical management of anemia involves addressing the underlying cause and managing the condition accordingly. Severe cases may require the replacement of lost or destroyed erythrocytes through packed red blood cell (PRBC) transfusions.

Gerontologic considerations underscore the prevalence and impact of anemia in elderly patients. It is the most common hematologic condition among this population and has significant implications for function and well-being. Studies have shown that anemia in the elderly is associated with increased fragility, reduced mobility and exercise capacity, higher risk of falls, cognitive decline, susceptibility to dementia and major depression, as well as lower skeletal muscle and bone density. These factors highlight the importance of early detection and management of anemia in geriatric patients to maintain their overall health and quality of life.

In the nursing process for patients with anemia, thorough assessment is crucial. This includes obtaining a detailed health history, conducting a comprehensive physical examination, and analyzing laboratory values. Patients should be questioned about the extent and type of symptoms experienced, their impact on daily life, medication history, alcohol consumption, and exercise habits. Family history of inherited anemias should also be explored. Nutritional assessment is essential, focusing on dietary habits that may contribute to nutritional deficiencies such as iron, vitamin B12, and folic acid. Monitoring relevant laboratory tests and assessing cardiac, gastrointestinal, and neurologic status are integral parts of the assessment process.

Nursing diagnosis for anemic patients may include fatigue due to decreased hemoglobin levels, altered nutrition resulting from inadequate intake of essential nutrients, and impaired tissue perfusion due to low hemoglobin and hematocrit levels. Noncompliance with prescribed therapy and potential complications such as heart failure, angina, paresthesias, and confusion should also be considered.

Goals for patient care should aim to reduce fatigue, ensure adequate nutrition and tissue perfusion, promote compliance with therapy, and prevent complications.

Nursing interventions focus on managing fatigue by assisting patients in prioritizing activities and maintaining a balance between activity and rest. Patients, especially those with chronic anemia, should be encouraged to engage in physical activity and exercise to prevent deconditioning.

Maintaining adequate nutrition is essential, and patients should be educated on healthy dietary choices, avoidance or limitation of alcohol intake, and cultural considerations related to nutrition. Nutritional supplements such as vitamins, iron, and folate should be discussed and prescribed as needed.

In ensuring adequate perfusion for patients with aplastic anemia, close monitoring of vital signs and pulse oximeter readings is essential. Medications, especially antihypertensives, may need adjustment or withholding based on individual patient responses. Administration of supplemental oxygen, transfusions, and intravenous fluids should be carried out according to physician orders.

Promoting compliance with prescribed therapy involves thorough patient education regarding medication purpose, administration instructions, potential side effects, and the importance of adherence. Patients should be assisted in integrating their therapeutic plan into their daily routines rather than merely receiving a list of instructions. Assistance in obtaining insurance coverage for expensive medications or exploring alternative means of access is crucial to ensure continuity of care.

Monitoring and managing complications is integral to patient care. Assessing for heart failure in patients with anemia and conducting neurologic assessments for those with known or suspected megaloblastic anemia are vital components of complication management.

Expected patient outcomes include reports of reduced fatigue, attainment and maintenance of adequate nutrition, maintenance of adequate perfusion, and minimal or no complications.

In nursing management of iron deficiency anemia, thorough assessment is crucial to identify signs of infection and bleeding, especially considering the vulnerability of patients with aplastic anemia to erythrocyte, leukocyte, and platelet deficiencies. Careful monitoring for side effects of therapy, particularly hypersensitivity reactions during administration of antithymocyte globulin (ATG), is essential. Long-term effects of cyclosporine therapy, including renal or liver dysfunction, hypertension, pruritus, visual impairment, tremor, and skin cancer, should be monitored for patients requiring prolonged treatment. Additionally, each new prescription should be meticulously assessed for potential drug interactions, as the metabolism of ATG can be altered by many other medications. Patient education is paramount to ensure understanding of the importance of not abruptly discontinuing immunosuppressive therapy.

Iron deficiency anemia typically occurs due to inadequate dietary iron intake for hemoglobin synthesis. It is the most prevalent type of anemia worldwide, affecting individuals of all age groups. Common causes in men and postmenopausal women include bleeding from ulcers, gastritis, inflammatory bowel disease, or gastrointestinal tumors. Premenopausal women commonly experience iron deficiency anemia due to menorrhagia (excessive menstrual bleeding) or inadequate iron supplementation during pregnancy. Chronic alcoholism can lead to iron deficiency anemia through chronic blood loss from the gastrointestinal tract. Other causes include iron malabsorption, as observed after gastrectomy or in individuals with celiac disease.

Clinical manifestations of iron deficiency anemia include typical symptoms of anemia, along with additional signs such as a smooth, sore tongue, brittle and ridged nails, and angular cheilitis (mouth ulceration) in more severe or prolonged cases. Diagnostic methods include bone marrow aspiration and laboratory tests to assess serum ferritin levels, blood cell count (hemoglobin, hematocrit, RBC count, mean corpuscular volume), serum iron level, and total iron-binding capacity.

Medical management involves identifying the underlying cause, which may include curable gastrointestinal cancer or uterine fibroids. Testing stool specimens for occult blood and performing periodic colonoscopies, endoscopies, or x-ray examinations of the gastrointestinal tract in individuals aged 50 years or older are recommended. Prescribed iron preparations (oral, intramuscular, or intravenous) should be administered, with patients advised to continue iron supplementation for 6 to 12 months. In cases where oral iron is not absorbed, poorly tolerated, or needed in large amounts, intramuscular or intravenous iron may be administered. Patients should be informed about potential side effects of iron supplementation, instructed on proper administration timing and techniques, and educated about dietary modifications to optimize iron absorption.

In the management of megaloblastic anemia resulting from deficiencies of vitamin B12 or folic acid, preventive education plays a crucial role, especially for menstruating and pregnant women who are at higher risk. Patient education should include guidance on foods rich in iron, such as organ meats, beans, leafy green vegetables, raisins, and molasses, to help improve iron levels. Patients should be advised to avoid taking antacids or dairy products with iron, as these can diminish iron absorption. Nutritional counseling should be provided for individuals with inadequate dietary intake to ensure they receive sufficient nutrients. Patients should be encouraged to continue iron therapy for the prescribed duration, typically 6 to 12 months, even after fatigue symptoms subside.

The pathophysiology of folic acid deficiency involves rapid depletion of folate stores in the body due to inadequate dietary intake, with alcohol consumption and chronic hemolytic anemias exacerbating the deficiency. Symptoms of folic acid and vitamin B12 deficiencies are similar and progressive, including weakness, fatigue, sore tongue, diarrhea, jaundice, vitiligo, premature graying, confusion, and paresthesias. Clinical manifestations may vary, with neurologic manifestations more common in vitamin B12 deficiency. Assessment and diagnostic findings include the Schilling test and laboratory tests to evaluate serum folate and vitamin B12 levels.

Medical management of folic acid deficiency includes increasing dietary intake of folic acid and administering 1 mg daily, with additional supplements as necessary. For vitamin B12 deficiency, oral supplements or monthly intramuscular injections of vitamin B12 are provided, depending on the cause of deficiency. Nursing management involves assessing patients for clinical manifestations, performing neurologic assessments, evaluating the need for assistive devices and therapy, ensuring safety, providing dietary guidance, and educating patients on diagnostic tests and compliance. It's crucial to address nutritional deficiencies comprehensively to manage megaloblastic anemia effectively.

In the management of sickle cell anemia, patient education is essential to ensure understanding of the chronicity of the disorder and the necessity of monthly vitamin B12 injections, even in the absence of symptoms. Patients should be instructed on self-administration of injections when appropriate, empowering them to take control of their treatment. Emphasis should be placed on the importance of ongoing medical follow-up and screening, particularly due to the increased risk of gastric carcinoma associated with gastric atrophy in pernicious anemia.

Sickle cell anemia is a severe hemolytic anemia resulting from the inheritance of the sickle hemoglobin (HbS) gene, which causes a defective hemoglobin molecule. The pathophysiology involves the assumption of a sickle shape by defective hemoglobin molecules when exposed to low oxygen tension, leading to obstruction of blood flow and tissue ischemia or infarction. Clinical manifestations vary and result from chronic hemolysis or thrombosis, including anemia, jaundice, bone marrow expansion, cardiac complications, organ thrombosis, and severe pain crises.

Diagnostic findings include low hematocrit levels and sickled cells on smear, confirmed by hemoglobin electrophoresis. Medical management focuses on symptom management and complication prevention. Treatment modalities include pharmacologic therapy, transfusion therapy, pulmonary function monitoring, and supportive care such as pain management, hydration, therapy, and counseling. Overall, a comprehensive approach is necessary to effectively manage sickle cell anemia and improve patient outcomes.

Nursing Process for Patient with Sickle Cell

In managing a patient experiencing a sickle cell crisis, the nursing process involves thorough assessment, diagnosis, planning, and intervention to address the patient's needs and prevent complications. Assessment includes questioning the patient about factors precipitating the crisis and measures taken to prevent it, along with a comprehensive examination of all body systems, particularly focusing on pain, swelling, fever, respiratory function, cardiac status, neurological signs, hydration status, and signs of infection. Monitoring of laboratory values, such as hemoglobin, hematocrit, and reticulocyte count, is crucial to track the patient's condition.

Nursing diagnoses may include acute pain related to tissue hypoxia, risk for infection, risk for powerlessness, and deficient knowledge regarding crisis prevention. Potential complications to be addressed include hypoxia, ischemia, infection, dehydration, cerebrovascular accident, anemia, renal failure, heart failure, pulmonary hypertension, impotence, poor compliance, and substance abuse.

Goals for the patient include pain relief, decreased incidence of crises, enhanced self-esteem and sense of power, and absence of complications. Nursing interventions focus on pain management, infection prevention, coping skills promotion, and patient education. Pain management strategies involve using the patient's subjective description and pain rating to guide analgesic administration, supporting and elevating swollen joints, teaching relaxation techniques, and implementing measures to preserve function. Infection prevention measures include monitoring for signs of infection, initiating antibiotics promptly, assessing for dehydration, and educating the patient about antibiotic therapy. Coping skills promotion involves enhancing pain management, focusing on patient strengths, providing opportunities for patient decision-making, and increasing knowledge about crisis prevention and management. Additionally, monitoring and managing potential complications are essential components of nursing care, requiring comprehensive measures tailored to the individual patient's needs.

Leg Ulcers

For leg ulcers, it's essential to protect the leg from trauma and contamination, utilizing scrupulous aseptic techniques to prevent nosocomial infections. Referring the patient to a wound–ostomy–a continence nurse can facilitate healing and provide assistance with prevention strategies.

In cases of priapism leading to impotence, patients should be taught to empty the bladder at the onset of the attack, engage in exercise, and take a warm bath. Patients should seek medical attention if an episode persists for more than three hours.

For chronic pain and substance abuse, emphasizing compliance with the prescribed treatment plan is crucial. Building trust with the patient through adequate management of acute pain during crisis episodes is essential. Encouraging continuity of care by receiving treatment from a single provider over time rather than rotating physicians and staff in an emergency department can be more beneficial. During crises, emergency department staff should contact the patient's primary health care provider for optimal management and establish written contracts with the patient to promote continuity of care.

Promoting home- and community-based care involves involving the patient and their family in teaching about the disease, treatment, assessment, and monitoring for complications. This includes education on vascular access device management and chelation therapy. Regular communication between healthcare providers, patients, and families is advised, along with providing guidelines on when to seek urgent care and offering follow-up care for patients with vascular access devices if necessary.

In evaluating patient outcomes, the expected results include reports of pain control, freedom from infection, an improved sense of control, increased knowledge about the disease process, and the absence of complications. Gerontologic considerations include recognizing that most abdominal aortic aneurysms occur in patients between 60 and 90 years of age, with rupture being likely in cases of coexisting hypertension and aneurysms wider than 6 cm.

Assessment of the Patient with Angina

Aortic aneurysms present various clinical manifestations depending on their location. In thoracic aortic aneurysms, symptoms may include constant, boring pain, dyspnea, cough, hoarseness, dilated superficial veins, edematous areas on the chest wall, cyanosis, and unequal pupils. Abdominal aortic aneurysms may be asymptomatic in about 60% of cases, with symptoms including abdominal pulsations, sensation of "heart beating" in the abdomen, and cyanosis with mottling of the toes if associated with thrombus. Dissecting aneurysms manifest with sudden, severe, and persistent tearing or ripping pain, along with pallor, sweating, tachycardia, and elevated blood pressure.

Diagnostic methods vary depending on the type of aneurysm. Thoracic aortic aneurysms are typically diagnosed using chest x-ray, CT angiography (CTA), and transesophageal echocardiography (TEE). Abdominal aortic aneurysms are diagnosed through palpation of a pulsatile mass in the upper abdomen, with duplex ultrasonography or CTA confirming the size, length, and location of the aneurysm. Dissecting aneurysms are diagnosed using arteriography, CTA, TEE, duplex ultrasonography, and magnetic resonance angiography (MRA).

Medical and surgical treatments vary based on the type of aneurysm. For ruptured aneurysms, surgery is performed immediately. Medical management includes strict blood pressure control, with systolic pressure maintained between 100 to 120 mm Hg using antihypertensive agents. Surgical management involves repairing abdominal aortic aneurysms more than 5.5 cm wide or those enlarging, typically through open surgical repair or endovascular grafting for infrarenal abdominal aortic aneurysms.

Nursing management encompasses preoperative and postoperative assessments, including monitoring pulmonary, cardiovascular, renal, and neurological status for complications such as arterial occlusion, hemorrhage, infection, ischemic bowel, renal failure, and impotence. It is essential to anticipate a rupture and recognize potential cardiovascular, cerebral, pulmonary, and renal impairments. The goal is to stabilize the patient medically before surgery and monitor them closely postoperatively for any signs of complications.

Assessment of Appendicitis in the Elderly

Gerontologic Considerations
Signs and symptoms in elderly patients may be atypical, resembling bowel obstruction or other conditions. Delayed presentation increases the risk of perforation due to delayed healthcare seeking behaviors.

Medical Management
Surgery, whether conventional or laparoscopic, is the primary treatment to prevent appendix rupture. Antibiotics and IV fluids are administered preoperatively to stabilize the patient.

Complications of Appendectomy
Perforation can lead to peritonitis, abscess formation, or portal pylephlebitis. Symptoms include fever, toxic appearance, and continued abdominal pain.

Nursing Management

Nursing goals involve pain relief, fluid balance maintenance, anxiety reduction, infection prevention, skin integrity maintenance, and optimal nutrition. Preoperative care includes IV line initiation, antibiotic administration, and nasogastric tube insertion if paralytic ileus is suspected. Postoperatively, patients are placed in a high Fowler's position, given analgesics, and gradually introduced to oral fluids and food.

Assessment and Management of Arterial Embolism and Arterial Thrombosis

Clinical Manifestations
Symptoms depend on embolus size, organ involved, and collateral circulation status. The six "P's—pain, pallor, pulselessness, paresthesia, poikilothermia, and paralysis—may be observed.

Medical Management
Heparin therapy followed by emergency embolectomy is initiated for acute embolic occlusion. Thrombolytic therapy may be considered in some cases, while anticoagulants are used to prevent thrombosis.

Nursing Management
Encourage leg movement to stimulate circulation and prevent stasis. Continuation of anticoagulants helps prevent further thrombus formation.

Understanding Arteriosclerosis and Atherosclerosis

Pathophysiology
Arteriosclerosis involves thickening of small arteries and arterioles, while atherosclerosis primarily affects large and medium-sized arteries, causing lipid accumulation and narrowing.

Risk Factors
Various factors contribute to atherosclerosis, including tobacco use, high fat intake, hypertension, diabetes, obesity, stress, lack of exercise, and elevated C-reactive protein.

Clinical Manifestations
Manifestations vary depending on the affected tissue or organ and can include angina, MI, transient ischemic attacks, stroke, hypertension, and peripheral artery disease.

Management

Management involves risk factor modification, exercise programs, medication therapy, and surgical procedures such as angioplasty and stent placement.

Nursing Care for Rheumatoid Arthritis

Clinical Manifestations
RA presents with joint pain, swelling, warmth, erythema, and loss of function. Joint deformities, fatigue, and systemic symptoms are common.

Assessment and Diagnostic Methods
Diagnosis is based on joint inflammation, laboratory findings, and extra-articular changes. Rheumatoid factor and erythrocyte sedimentation rate are often elevated.

Medical Management
Treatment includes education, medication therapy, physical and occupational therapy, and surgical interventions in severe cases.

Nursing Management
Nursing care focuses on pain relief, fatigue management, mobility promotion, self-care

facilitation, complication monitoring, and patient education for home care continuation.

Promoting Home- and Community-Based Care

#Teaching Patients Self-Care
Patient education covers disease management, medication adherence, lifestyle modifications, and safety measures at home.

Continuing Care
Referral to home care services may be necessary for patients with limited function. Assessing the home environment, addressing barriers to compliance, and providing ongoing support are essential for optimal patient outcomes.

Asthma

Introduction

Asthma is a chronic inflammatory disease of the airways characterized by hyperresponsiveness, mucosal edema, and mucus production.

Epidemiology and Risk Factors

Asthma, the most common chronic disease of childhood, can develop at any age. Risk factors include family history, allergies, and chronic exposure to irritants or allergens.

Clinical Manifestations

Symptoms include cough, dyspnea, wheezing, and chest tightness, often worse at night or in the early morning.

Types and Complications

Exercise-induced asthma and status are severe forms. Allergic reactions and eczema may accompany asthma.

Assessment and Diagnosis

History, physical exam, pulmonary function tests, and blood tests aid in diagnosis during acute episodes.

Medical Management

Pharmacologic therapy includes short-acting beta2-adrenergic agonists, corticosteroids, and leukotriene modifiers.

Nursing Management

Nursing care focuses on assessing respiratory status, administering medications, and promoting patient and family education.

Home and Community Care

Patients are taught self-care, including medication use, trigger avoidance, and peak-flow monitoring. Follow-up appointments and community support groups are emphasized.

Status Asthmaticus

This severe and persistent form requires immediate medical intervention, including oxygen therapy, bronchodilators, and possibly mechanical ventilation.

Conclusion

Asthma management involves a multidisciplinary approach focusing on symptom control, patient education, and prevention of exacerbations.

Benign Prostatic Hyperplasia and Prostatectomy

Introduction
Benign prostatic hyperplasia (BPH) involves the enlargement of the prostate gland, obstructing urine outflow.

Clinical Manifestations
- Hesitancy, increased frequency of urination, nocturia, urgency.
- Decreased urinary stream volume and force, interruption, dribbling.
- Sensation of incomplete bladder emptying, acute urinary retention, recurrent UTIs.
- Fatigue, anorexia, nausea, vomiting, pelvic discomfort, azotemia, renal failure.

Assessment and Diagnostic Methods
- Digital rectal examination, health history.
- Urinalysis, prostate-specific antigen (PSA) level, urinary flow-rate recording, post void residual (PVR) urine.

- Urodynamic studies, urethrocystoscopy, ultrasound, complete blood studies.

Medical Management
- Immediate catheterization if unable to avoid, "watchful waiting," pharmacologic management, hormonal manipulation, surgical management (minimally invasive therapy, surgical resection).

Nursing Management
- Similar to "Nursing Process: The Patient Undergoing Prostatectomy" under "Cancer of the Prostate."

Conclusion
Benign prostatic hyperplasia requires a comprehensive approach including medical and nursing management strategies.

Neoplasms of the Musculoskeletal System

Introduction
Neoplasms of the musculoskeletal system encompass various types, including benign and malignant tumors.

Types
- Benign Bone Tumors: Slow-growing, encapsulated, producing few symptoms.
- Malignant Bone Tumors: Primary tumors arising from connective and supportive tissue cells, metastatic tumors.
- Soft Tissue Sarcomas: Liposarcoma, fibrosarcoma, rhabdomyosarcoma.

Clinical Manifestations
- Asymptomatic or pain, varying degrees of disability, weight loss, malaise, fever, spinal metastasis.
- Symptoms may vary depending on tumor type and location.

Assessment and Diagnostic Findings
- Imaging studies (CT scan, bone scan, MRI), biochemical assays, surgical biopsy.

Medical Management
- Surgical excision, radiation, chemotherapy, limb-sparing procedures.
- Palliative treatment for metastatic bone cancer.

Nursing Management
- Pain management, patient education, emotional support, rehabilitation.

Conclusion
Neoplasms of the musculoskeletal system require a multidisciplinary approach for effective management and care.

Bowel Obstruction, Large

Introduction
Large bowel obstruction impedes the flow of intestinal contents, leading to severe distention and potential complications.

Clinical Manifestations
- Constipation, blood loss in stool, weakness, weight loss, anorexia, abdominal distention, crampy lower abdominal pain, fecal vomiting, shock.

Assessment and Diagnostic Methods
- Symptoms assessment, imaging studies (abdominal x-ray, CT scan, MRI).

Medical Management

Nonpharmacologic Interventions
- Bed Rest and Activity Modification: Limited to 1 to 2 days for severe pain, emphasizing gradual return to activities.

- Superficial Heat and Spinal Manipulation:Effective for pain relief.
- Cognitive-Behavioral Therapy and Exercise Regimens:Effective for chronic low back pain.
- Patient Education: Emphasizes activity modification and avoidance of exacerbating movements.

Pharmacologic Therapy
- Acute Low Back Pain:Nonprescription analgesics, NSAIDs, and prescription muscle relaxants.
- Chronic Low Back Pain:Tricyclic antidepressants, opioids, tramadol, benzodiazepines, and gabapentin.

Nursing Management

Assessment:
- Pain Description and History:Location, severity, duration, characteristics, radiation, and impact on lifestyle.

- Physical Examination: Posture, gait, spinal curves, muscle spasm, tenderness, limitations in movement, nerve involvement, and obesity.
- Response to Analgesic Agents: Monitoring effectiveness and side effects.

Interventions
- Activity Limitation: Initial rest for severe pain.
- Bedding and Positioning:Firm mattress, lumbar flexion support, and proper techniques for getting out of bed.
- Exercise Program: Gradual resumption of activities, including low-stress aerobic and conditioning exercises.
- Posture Improvement:Emphasizing good body mechanics and avoidance of lumbar strain and twisting.

Bowel Obstruction, Small

Pathophysiology
- Location and Accumulation: Most occur in the small intestine; accumulation of intestinal contents, fluid, and gas above obstruction.
- Effects of Distention: Abdominal distention, decreased venous and arteriolar capillary pressure, edema, congestion, necrosis, and potential rupture or perforation.
- Clinical Manifestations: Crampy, colicky pain, blood and mucus in stool, vomiting, and signs of dehydration.

Assessment and Diagnostic Findings
- Symptoms: Crampy pain, vomiting, dehydration.
- Imaging Studies: Abnormal quantities of gas and/or fluid in intestines.
- Laboratory Studies: Electrolytes and complete blood count showing dehydration and possibly infection.

Medical Management
- Decompression: Nasogastric or small bowel tube for partial obstruction; surgical intervention for complete or strangulated obstruction.
- Surgical Treatment: Depends on cause (e.g., hernia repair); IV therapy before surgery to replace fluids and electrolytes.

Nursing Management
- Nonsurgical Patient: Maintain nasogastric tube function, assess output, monitor fluid and electrolyte balance, evaluate nutritional status, and assess improvement.
- Monitoring: Discrepancies in intake/output, worsening pain or distention, increased nasogastric output.
- Preparation for Surgery: If a patient's condition does not improve with conservative management.

Brain Abscess

Pathophysiology
- Formation: Collection of infectious material within brain tissue, commonly caused by bacteria.
- Routes of Infection: Hematologic spread, penetrating head injury, or surgical procedures.
- Prevention: Prompt treatment of otitis media, mastoiditis, rhinosinusitis, dental infections, and systemic infections.

Clinical Manifestations
- Symptoms: Headache (worse in the morning), fever, vomiting, focal neurologic deficits, increased intracranial pressure (ICP).

Assessment and Diagnostic Methods:
- Neuroimaging Studies: MRI or CT scanning to identify size and location of abscess.
- Aspiration: Guided by CT or MRI to culture and identify infectious organisms.

- Additional Tests: Blood cultures, chest x-ray, EEG.

Medical Management
- Treatment Modalities: Antimicrobial therapy, surgical incision or aspiration, corticosteroids to reduce cerebral edema, anti seizure medications.
- Monitoring: Abscess resolution with CT scans.

Nursing Management
- Supportive Care: Nursing interventions to support medical treatment, patient teaching on neurosurgical procedures, assessment of family coping and support needs.

Bronchiectasis

Definition and Etiology
- Chronic, Irreversible Dilation: Bronchi and bronchioles affected, separate from COPD.
- Causes: Airway obstruction, infections, genetic disorders (e.g., cystic fibrosis), abnormal host defense, idiopathic factors.

Clinical Manifestations
- Chronic Symptoms: Persistent cough, copious purulent sputum, hemoptysis, clubbing of fingers, recurrent pulmonary infections.

Assessment and Diagnosis
- Diagnostic Clue: Prolonged history of productive cough with negative tubercle bacilli.
- Diagnostic Tool: CT scan for definitive diagnosis.

Medical Management
- Treatment Objectives: Promote bronchial drainage, prevent/control infection.

- Interventions: Chest physiotherapy, postural drainage, expectorants, bronchoscopy for secretion removal.

Chronic Bronchitis

Definition and Pathophysiology
- Definition: Cough and sputum production for 3 months in consecutive years, related to airway irritation and inflammation.
- Pathophysiology: Chronic irritation leads to increased mucus production, thickening of bronchial walls, and reduced ciliary function.

Clinical Manifestations
- Symptoms: Chronic cough, increased mucus production, exacerbated by environmental pollutants.
- Exacerbations: Common during winter months due to increased viral and bacterial infections.

Nursing Management
- Preventive Measures: Smoking cessation, vaccination against influenza and pneumococcal pneumonia.
- Treatment Approaches: Antibiotics, bronchodilators, surgery (infrequently).

- Preoperative Preparation: Postural drainage, suction through bronchoscope, antibacterial therapy.

Buerger's Disease (Thromboangiitis Obliterans)

Definition and Epidemiology
- Definition: Recurring inflammation of intermediate and small arteries and veins of extremities.
- Demographics: Predominantly affects men aged 20-35, associated with heavy tobacco use.

Clinical Manifestations
- Symptoms: Pain (bilateral and symmetric), claudication, burning pain, cold sensitivity, color changes, paresthesia, ulceration, gangrene.

Assessment and Diagnosis
- Diagnostic Methods: Segmental limb blood pressures, duplex ultrasonography, contrast angiography.

Medical Management
- Objectives: Improve circulation, prevent disease progression, protect extremities.

- Interventions: Tobacco cessation, sympathetic block, debridement, amputation if necessary.

Nursing Management
- Supportive Care: Similar to peripheral arterial occlusive disease management.
- Preventive Measures: Smoking cessation, monitoring for complications, providing emotional support.

Assessing Patient and Family Understanding and Coping

- Assessment: Understand patient and family comprehension of burn injury, coping mechanisms, family dynamics, and anxiety levels. Provide tailored support and explanations.
- Interventions: Offer pain relief and administer anti anxiety medications if necessary.

Monitoring and Managing Potential Complications

- Acute Respiratory Failure: Watch for dyspnea, changes in respiratory patterns, monitor oxygen saturation and CO_2 levels, perform chest x-rays, and assess for cerebral hypoxia. Be prepared to assist with intubation or escharotomy.
- Distributive Shock: Monitor for signs of shock and progressive edema. Administer fluid resuscitation and closely monitor fluid status.
- Acute Renal Failure: Monitor urine output and quality, blood urea nitrogen (BUN), and creatinine levels. Administer increased fluids as prescribed.
- Compartment Syndrome: Assess peripheral pulses hourly, evaluate neurovascular status, and be prepared to assist with escharotomies.
- Paralytic Ileus: Maintain nasogastric tube and monitor for distention and bowel sounds.
- Curling's Ulcer: Assess gastric aspirate for blood and pH, monitor stools for occult blood, and administer antacids and histamine blockers as prescribed.

Nursing Management: Acute Phase

Assessment

- Focus on hemodynamic alterations, wound healing, pain, psychosocial responses, and early complication detection.
- Measure vital signs frequently, with respiratory and fluid status a priority.
- Monitor peripheral pulses, fluid intake/output, and cardiac rhythm closely.

Interventions

- Restore fluid balance by monitoring IV and oral fluid intake and output, using IV infusion pumps, and reporting changes promptly.
- Prevent infection through maintaining a clean environment, scrutinizing wounds, practicing aseptic techniques, and educating patients on wound care.
- Maintain adequate nutrition by slowly initiating oral fluids, collaborating with

dietitians, documenting caloric intake, and providing nutritional supplements if needed.
- Promote skin integrity through wound assessment, supporting patients during wound care, and coordinating dressing changes.
- Relieve pain and discomfort by frequent assessment, administering analgesics, teaching relaxation techniques, and promoting comfort measures during healing.
- Promote physical mobility to prevent complications of immobility and encourage early sitting and ambulation.
- Strengthen coping strategies by assisting patients in developing effective coping mechanisms, involving patients in care decisions, and providing support for patients and families.
- Monitor and manage potential complications such as heart failure, pulmonary edema, sepsis, acute respiratory failure, and visceral damage.

Nursing Process: Rehabilitation Phase

Assessment

- Early Assessment: Gather information on a patient's background, including education, occupation, leisure activities, cultural and religious affiliations, and family dynamics.
- Psychosocial Assessment: Evaluate self-concept, emotional response to injury and hospitalization, intellectual functioning, previous hospitalizations, pain response, and sleep patterns.
- Ongoing Assessments: Continuously monitor rehabilitation goals, range of motion, functional abilities, signs of skin breakdown, neuropathies, activity tolerance, and skin healing.
- Comprehensive Assessment: Document participation and self-care abilities in various activities and maintain continuous assessment for early complication detection.

Diagnosis

- Nursing Diagnoses: Address activity intolerance, disturbed body image, and deficient knowledge of postdischarge care and recovery needs.
- Collaborative Problems: Address inadequate psychological adaptation to burn injury.

Planning and Goals

- Establish goals for increased participation in activities of daily living (ADLs), improved understanding of injury and treatment, adjustment to changes in body image and self-concept, and prevention of complications.

Nursing Interventions

Promoting Activity Tolerance

- Ensure uninterrupted sleep periods and administer hypnotic agents if needed.
- Communicate care plans to family and caregivers.

- Relieve pain, prevent fever, and monitor fatigue to conserve energy.
- Incorporate physical therapy exercises to maintain mobility.
- Schedule diversion activities to increase tolerance for activity.

Improving Body Image and Self-Concept

- Listen to the patient's concerns and provide realistic support.
- Assess psychosocial reactions and provide coping strategies.
- Support patients through small gestures and provide information on cosmetic resources.

Monitoring and Managing Potential Complications

- Contractures: Provide early and aggressive physical and occupational therapy, and support surgery if necessary.
- Impaired Psychological Adaptation: Refer for psychological or psychiatric support as needed.

Promoting Home- and Community-Based Care

- Educate patients and families on wound care, complication prevention, pain management, and nutrition.
- Provide written instructions and identify abnormal signs requiring physician notification.
- Assist in planning continued care and refer to home care resources if needed.

Evaluation

Expected Patient Outcomes

- Demonstrates increased activity tolerance for daily activities.
- Adapts to altered body image.
- Exhibits knowledge of required self-care and follow-up care.
- Experiences no complications.

Promoting Nutrition

Teaching Strategies
- Educate patients to avoid unpleasant sights, odors, and sounds during mealtime.
- Recommend preferred high-calorie, high-protein foods respecting cultural preferences.
- Encourage adequate fluid intake, limiting fluids during meals.
- Suggest smaller, frequent meals.
- Create a relaxed, quiet mealtime environment with social interaction.
- Advocate for nutritional supplements and high-protein snacks between meals.
- Emphasize oral hygiene and pain relief measures to enhance meal enjoyment.
- Manage nausea, vomiting, and anxiety during meals.
- Collaborate for enteral tube feedings or appetite stimulants if prescribed.
- Discourage pressure from family and friends regarding eating habits.

- Assess and address contributing factors to nutritional issues.

Relieving Pain

Multidisciplinary Approach
- Employ a team approach to pain management for optimal quality of life.
- Validate patient's pain experiences and offer assistance in alleviating discomfort.
- Involve patients and family in pain management decisions.
- Educate to correct misconceptions about pain management.

Pain Relief Strategies
- Encourage previously successful pain relief strategies.
- Teach new pain relief techniques such as distraction, imagery, and relaxation.
- Address factors contributing to pain and implement appropriate interventions.

Decreasing Fatigue

Understanding Fatigue
- Explain fatigue as a common, temporary side effect of cancer and its treatments.
- Help patients organize activities to conserve energy.
- Assist in reallocating responsibilities to conserve energy.
- Support adequate nutrition, hydration, and exercise.
- Encourage relaxation techniques and light exercise.

Improving Body Image and Self-Esteem

Tailored Approach
- Assess a patient's body image concerns and self-esteem levels.
- Validate patient's concerns and encourage continued participation in activities.
- Assist in self-care activities and appearance management.

- Address concerns about altered sexuality and refer to specialists if needed.

Assisting in Grieving

Emotional Support
- Encourage expression of fears and concerns.
- Involve patients and families in care decisions.
- Maintain regular communication and emotional closeness.
- Facilitate spiritual support as desired.
- Support the grieving process at patient and family's pace.

Monitoring and Managing Potential Complications

Managing Infection
- Assess for signs of infection and report promptly.
- Educate on infection prevention measures.
- Ensure strict hand hygiene and aseptic techniques.

- Minimize invasive procedures and urinary catheterization.

Managing Septic Shock
- Monitor for signs of septic shock and provide prompt treatment.
- Educate on signs of septicemia and prevention measures.

Managing Bleeding and Hemorrhage
- Monitor platelet count and assess for bleeding.
- Educate on minimizing bleeding risks and provide interventions.
- Institute bed rest and platelet transfusions as needed.

Promoting Home- and Community-Based Care

Teaching Patients Self-Care
- Provide information and support for home care needs.
- Discuss treatment side effects and management strategies.

- Identify learning needs and provide ongoing support.

Continuing Care
- Refer for home care services and assess a patient's physical status.
- Coordinate care among healthcare providers and community resources.
- Ensure follow-up visits and evaluate patient progress.

Nursing Management Related to Treatment

Cancer Surgery
- Conduct preoperative assessments and provide emotional support.
- Monitor postoperative responses and manage complications.
- Provide postoperative teaching and discharge planning.

Radiation Therapy
- Address patient's concerns and assess treatment side effects.
- Provide supportive care and educate on self-care practices.

Chemotherapy
- Monitor nutritional and fluid status and assess for complications.
- Administer chemotherapy and monitor for adverse effects.
- Educate on symptom management and precautions.

Bone Marrow Transplantation
- Conduct comprehensive assessments before BMT.
- Monitor for acute toxicities and provide ongoing support.
- Assess for graft-versus-host disease and late effects.

Hyperthermia
- Educate patients on the procedure and manage adverse effects.
- Provide local skin care at hyperthermic probe sites.

Biologic Response Modifiers
- Assess patient and family needs and monitor for therapeutic and adverse effects.

Cancer of the Bladder

Clinical Manifestations
- Common symptoms include painless hematuria and urinary tract infections.
- Any alteration in voiding or urine should be evaluated.

Assessment and Diagnostic Methods
- Biopsies and imaging studies aid in diagnosis.
- New diagnostic tools are under study.

Medical Management
- Treatment depends on tumor grade and stage.
- Surgical options include TUR, cystectomy, or trimodal therapy.
- Pharmacologic therapy includes chemotherapy and intravesical BCG.

Radiation Therapy
- Used preoperatively or in combination with surgery.

- Hydrostatic therapy and formalin installations can relieve symptoms.

Nursing Management
- Provide comprehensive care similar to cancer surgery, radiation, and chemotherapy.
- Monitor for complications and provide support.

Cancer of the Breast

Risk Factors
- Gender, age, family history, and genetic mutations increase risk.
- Hormonal factors and lifestyle choices also play a role.

Prevention Strategies
- Surveillance, chemoprevention, and prophylactic mastectomy may be considered.

Clinical Manifestations
- Breast lesions are typically nontender with irregular borders.
- Advanced signs include skin changes and nipple retraction.

Assessment and Diagnostic Methods
- Biopsy and staging help determine treatment options.
- Imaging studies and blood work aid in diagnosis and staging.

Medical Management
- Treatment options include surgery, radiation, chemotherapy, and hormonal therapy.
- Management is tailored based on tumor characteristics and patient preferences.

NURSING PROCESS: THE PATIENT UNDERGOING SURGERY FOR BREAST CANCER

Assessment

- Health History: Gather a patient's medical background.
- Reaction to Diagnosis: Assess patient's response and coping abilities.

Diagnosis

Preoperative Nursing Diagnoses:
- Deficient Knowledge about surgical treatments.
- Anxiety related to cancer diagnosis.
- Fear related to treatments and body image changes.
- Risk for ineffective coping.
- Decisional conflict about treatment options.

Postoperative Nursing Diagnoses:

- Pain and discomfort post-surgery.
- Disturbed sensory perception.
- Disturbed body image.
- Risk for impaired adjustment.
- Self-care deficit.
- Risk for sexual dysfunction.
- Deficient knowledge about drain management, arm exercises, and hand care.

Collaborative Problems/Potential Complications:
- Lymphedema.
- Hematoma/Seroma.
- Infection.

Planning and Goals

Major goals include increased knowledge, reduced fear, improved coping, decision-making ability, pain management, sexual function, and absence of complications.

Preoperative Nursing Interventions

- Provide education about treatments.

- Prepare patients for surgery.
- Inform about decreased mobility and demonstrate exercises.
- Reassure about pain management.

Postoperative Nursing Interventions

- Relieve pain and discomfort.
- Manage postoperative sensations.
- Promote positive body image.
- Support coping and adjustment.
- Improve sexual function.
- Monitor and manage complications.

Home- and Community-Based Care

- Teach self-care.
- Provide follow-up support.
- Reinforce earlier teaching.
- Encourage follow-up visits.

Evaluation

Expected outcomes include knowledge about diagnosis, coping ability, pain management, clean incision, and absence of complications.

- Assess psychosocial support.

Diagnosis

- Anxiety related to cancer diagnosis and surgery.
- Disturbed body image.
- Pain.
- Deficient knowledge.

Collaborative Problems/Potential Complications

- Hemorrhage.
- Deep vein thrombosis.
- Bladder dysfunction.
- Infection.

Planning and Goals

Goals include anxiety relief, improved body image, pain management, increased knowledge, and absence of complications.

Nursing Interventions

- Relieve anxiety.
- Improve body image.
- Relieve pain.
- Monitor and manage complications.

Home- and Community-Based Care

- Tailor information according to the patient's needs.
- Stress the importance of self-care.
- Encourage gradual resumption of activities.
- Reinforce follow-up appointments.

Evaluation

Expected outcomes include decreased anxiety, improved body image, minimal pain, understanding of self-care, and absence of complications.

COLORECTAL CANCER

Clinical Manifestations:
- Changes in bowel habits.
- Passage of blood in stools.
- Anemia, anorexia, weight loss, fatigue.

Assessment and Diagnostic Methods:
- Examination, fecal occult blood testing, imaging, CEA studies.

Gerontologic Considerations:
- Incidence increases with age.
- Symptoms are often insidious.

Medical Management:
- Treatment depends on the disease stage.
- Surgery, chemotherapy, radiation, and supportive therapy.

Surgical Management

- Primary treatment for most cases.

- Type of surgery depends on the tumor location and size.

NURSING PROCESS: THE PATIENT UNDERGOING HYSTERECTOMY

Assessment

- Health History: Obtain comprehensive medical background.
- Physical Examination: Perform thorough physical and pelvic examination.
- Psychosocial Assessment: Gather data on a patient's emotional support and responses.

Diagnosis

Nursing Diagnoses:
- Anxiety related to cancer diagnosis, fear of pain, loss of femininity, or childbearing potential.
- Disturbed body image related to altered fertility, fears about sexuality, and relationships.
- Pain related to surgery and adjuvant therapy.
- Deficient knowledge of perioperative aspects and self-care.

Collaborative Problems/Potential Complications:
- Hemorrhage.
- Deep vein thrombosis.
- Bladder dysfunction.
- Infection.

Planning and Goals

Major goals include anxiety relief, body image improvement, pain management, increased self-care knowledge, and absence of complications.

Nursing Interventions

- Relieving Anxiety:
  - Acknowledge the patient's feelings and allow expression.
  - Explain pre- and postoperative procedures thoroughly.

- Improving Body Image:

- Assess a patient's feelings about surgery, diagnosis, and prognosis.
- Address concerns about fertility, femininity, and sexual relations.
- Educate about sexual satisfaction and comfort.

- Relieving Pain:
  - Assess pain intensity and administer analgesics.
  - Encourage gradual resumption of food and fluids intake.
  - Apply heat or insert a rectal tube for abdominal distention.

- Monitoring and Managing Complications:
  - Monitor perineal pads, vital signs, and abdominal dressings for hemorrhage.
  - Apply compression stockings and encourage early ambulation for deep vein thrombosis.
  - Monitor urinary output and encourage voiding for bladder dysfunction.

Promoting Home- and Community-Based Care

- Teaching Patients Self-Care:
  - Customize information according to the patient's needs.
  - Instruct on daily incision checks, adequate intake, and activity resumption.
  - Emphasize avoiding specific activities and reporting any abnormal symptoms promptly.

- Continuing Care:
  - Follow up with patients via telephone to address concerns and progress.
  - Remind patients about postoperative appointments and hormone therapy discussion if ovaries were removed.

Evaluation

Expected outcomes include decreased anxiety, improved body image, minimal pain, understanding of self-care, and absence of complications.

NURSING PROCESS: THE PATIENT WITH COLORECTAL CANCER

Assessment

- Health History:
  - Fatigue, abdominal or rectal pain.
  - Past and present elimination patterns, stool characteristics.
  - History of inflammatory bowel disease (IBD), colorectal polyps, family history of colorectal disease, and current medications.
  - Dietary patterns, including fat and fiber intake, alcohol consumption, smoking history, weight loss, weakness, and fatigue.

- Physical Examination:
  - Auscultate abdomen for bowel sounds.
  - Palpate for tenderness, distention, and masses.
  - Inspect stool for blood.

Diagnosis

Nursing Diagnoses:
- Imbalanced nutrition: less than body requirements.
- Risk for deficient fluid volume.
- Anxiety related to surgery and cancer diagnosis.
- Risk for ineffective therapeutic regimen management.
- Impaired skin integrity.
- Disturbed body image.
- Ineffective sexuality patterns.

Collaborative Problems/Potential Complications:
- Intraperitoneal infection.
- Complete large bowel obstruction.
- Gastrointestinal bleeding and hemorrhage.
- Bowel perforation.
- Peritonitis, abscess, sepsis.

Planning and Goals

Major goals include optimal nutrition, fluid balance, anxiety reduction, learning about diagnosis and self-care, tissue healing, peristomal skin protection, colostomy management, expression of feelings, and complication prevention.

Nursing Interventions

Preparing Patient for Surgery:
  - Provide high-calorie, high-protein diet or parenteral nutrition.
  - Administer prescribed medications and bowel preparations.
  - Monitor intake and output, IV fluids, and electrolyte balance.
  - Observe signs of hypovolemia, obstruction, or perforation.
  - Educate about diagnosis, surgery, postoperative care, wound, and ostomy care.

Providing Emotional Support:
  - Assess anxiety level and coping mechanisms.
  - Teach relaxation techniques, arrange spiritual meetings.
  - Facilitate discussions with healthcare providers.

Maintaining Optimal Nutrition:
 - Educate about healthy diet, individualized to avoid exacerbating symptoms.
 - Advise on fluid intake and avoidance of odor and gas-inducing foods.

Maintaining Fluid and Electrolyte Balance:
 - Administer antiemetics, restrict fluids to prevent vomiting.
 - Monitor electrolytes, hydration status, vital signs.

Supporting a Positive Body Image:
 - Encourage expression of feelings and concerns.
 - Provide a supportive environment and attitude.
 - Refer to appropriate support services.

Monitoring and Managing Complications:
 - Monitor for and report complications, administer antibiotics as prescribed.

- Assess wound and stoma, provide appropriate care.
- Educate on home care, complication recognition, and when to seek medical help.

Promoting Home- and Community-Based Care

Teaching Patients Self-Care:
- Provide tailored information to patients and families.
- Educate on ostomy care, dietary restrictions, medication management.
- Instruct on recognizing and managing complications.

Evaluation

Expected outcomes include maintaining nutrition and fluid balance, reduced anxiety, knowledge acquisition, wound and stoma care, expression of feelings, and complication-free recovery.

Nursing Process: The Patient Undergoing Laryngectomy

Assessment
- Health History: Assess physical, psychosocial, and spiritual domains.
- Symptoms: Evaluate for hoarseness, sore throat, dyspnea, dysphagia, or throat pain.
- Head and Neck Examination: Palpate for swelling, nodularity, or adenopathy.
- Functional Assessment: Evaluate ability to hear, see, read, and write.
- Psychological Status: Assess coping methods pre- and postoperatively.

Diagnosis
Nursing Diagnoses: Based on assessment data, diagnoses may include:
- Deficient knowledge about surgery and postoperative care.
- Anxiety and depression related to cancer diagnosis and surgery.

- Ineffective airway clearance due to surgical alterations.
- Impaired verbal communication due to laryngeal removal.
- Imbalanced nutrition due to swallowing difficulties.
- Disturbed body image and self-esteem due to surgery.
- Self-care deficit related to pain and weakness.

Collaborative Problems/Potential Complications
- Respiratory distress, hemorrhage, infection, aspiration, tracheostomal stenosis.

Planning and Goals
- Knowledge about treatment, reduced anxiety, maintenance of patent airway, effective communication, optimal nutrition, improved self-care, absence of complications.

Nursing Interventions
Teaching Preoperatively:
- Clarify misconceptions, provide educational materials.

- Explain potential outcomes and rehabilitation programs.
- Teach coughing, breathing exercises.

Reducing Anxiety and Depression:
- Allow expression of feelings, arrange peer visits.

Maintaining Airway:
- Positioning, observation for respiratory distress, encouraging coughing and deep breathing.

Promoting Alternative Communication:
- Work with speech therapists, provide communication aids.

Promoting Nutrition and Hydration:
- Maintain NPO status, start oral feedings gradually.

Improving Self-Concept:
- Encourage expression of feelings, refer to support groups.

Monitoring and Managing Complications:
- Monitor for signs of respiratory distress, hemorrhage, infection, aspiration, and stenosis.

Promoting Home- and Community-Based Care: Teaching Patients Self-Care
- Provide discharge instructions, assess readiness to learn.
- Instruct on tracheostomy care, nutrition, hygiene, and precautions.
- Encourage regular follow-up visits and health promotion activities.

Evaluation
- Expected outcomes include adequate knowledge, reduced anxiety, clear airway, effective communication, adequate nutrition, improved self-concept, absence of complications, adherence to rehabilitation and home care program.

Teaching Strategies for Patient and Family:

Prevention of Skin Breakdown and Symptom Management:
- Teach strategies for preventing skin breakdown and alleviating pain, pruritus, and anorexia.
- Provide instruction on Patient-Controlled Analgesia (PCA), Total Parenteral Nutrition (TPN), and dietary modifications, including pancreatic enzymes for malabsorption and hyperglycemia.
- Emphasize the importance of monitoring serum glucose levels for patients with pancreatic islet tumors.

Palliative Care Discussion:
- Discuss palliative care options with the patient and family to manage discomfort and support end-of-life decisions.

Instruction for Family on Reporting Changes:
- Instruct family members on recognizing and reporting changes in the patient's condition to the physician promptly.

Referral and Discharge Planning:
- Refer the patient for home care assistance to address problems, discomfort, and psychological effects.
- Coordinate discharge to a long-term care facility, ensuring communication with staff regarding prior teaching and care needs.

Continued Care and Monitoring:

Prostate Cancer Overview:
- Discuss the prevalence of prostate cancer, risk factors, and common clinical manifestations.
- Explain diagnostic methods, including digital rectal examination and prostate-specific antigen (PSA) testing.

Medical Management:
- Describe various treatment options based on patient factors and disease characteristics, such as radical prostatectomy, radiation therapy, hormone therapy, chemotherapy, and other interventions.

Nursing Process for Patient Undergoing Prostatectomy

Assessment and Diagnosis:
- Conduct a comprehensive assessment focusing on urinary function and impact on the patient's lifestyle.
- Identify preoperative nursing diagnoses related to anxiety, acute pain, and knowledge deficit.
- Anticipate potential postoperative nursing diagnoses, including acute pain and deficient knowledge.

Planning and Goals:
- Establish preoperative goals to reduce anxiety and educate the patient about their condition and upcoming surgery.
- Set postoperative goals for fluid balance, pain relief, self-care, and complication prevention.

Nursing Interventions:

- Implement interventions to reduce anxiety, alleviate discomfort, and provide preoperative education.
- Monitor fluid balance, administer pain relief measures, and manage potential complications postoperatively.

Patient Education and Home Care:

Self-Care Teaching Strategies:
- Educate the patient and family on managing drainage systems, monitoring urinary output, wound care, and complication prevention.
- Instruct on recognizing signs and symptoms requiring medical attention, performing perineal exercises, and addressing sexual dysfunction.

Continuing Care and Evaluation:
- Arrange for home care services as needed and emphasize the importance of continued bladder control recovery.
- Evaluate patient outcomes, including reduced anxiety, pain relief, self-care abilities, absence of

complications, and understanding of sexual function changes.

NURSING PROCESS: THE PATIENT WITH MALIGNANT MELANOMA

Assessment:
- Patient History: Inquire about pruritus, tenderness, and pain, unique to malignant melanoma.
- Skin Examination: Use a magnifying lens to check for irregularities and changes in moles.
- Signs of Malignancy: Look for asymmetry, irregular border, variegated color, and large diameter (ABCDs of moles).
- Common Sites: Pay attention to areas like the back, legs, face, and fingernails.

Diagnosis:
- Nursing Diagnoses: Include acute pain, anxiety, depression, and deficient knowledge about melanoma.
- Collaborative Problems: Address metastasis and infection of surgical sites.

Planning and Goals:
- Patient Goals: Aim for pain relief, reduced anxiety and depression, increased knowledge of melanoma signs, and absence of complications.

Nursing Interventions:
- Pain Management: Administer appropriate analgesics and promote comfort.
- Anxiety Reduction: Offer support, allow expression of feelings, and provide information and resources for coping.
- Complication Monitoring: Educate about treatment, potential side effects, and expected outcomes. Encourage hope while being realistic.

Evaluation:
- Expected Outcomes: Relief of pain, reduced anxiety, understanding of melanoma detection and prevention, and absence of complications.

NURSING PROCESS: THE PATIENT WITH STOMACH CANCER

Assessment:
- Dietary History: Elicit dietary intake and assess weight loss and eating habits.
- Symptom Assessment: Identify pain, early satiety, and anorexia.
- Psychosocial Assessment: Evaluate coping skills, emotional resources, and family support.

Diagnosis:
- Nursing Diagnoses: Address anxiety, imbalanced nutrition, pain, anticipatory grieving, and deficient knowledge.

Planning and Goals:
- Patient Goals: Strive for reduced anxiety, optimal nutrition, pain relief, and adjustment to lifestyle changes.

Nursing Interventions:

- Anxiety Reduction: Create a relaxed atmosphere, encourage family support, and provide information about procedures and treatments.
- Nutritional Support: Encourage small, frequent meals and monitor intake, output, and weight.
- Pain Management: Administer analgesics, suggest nonpharmacologic pain relief methods, and provide psychological support.

Promoting Home- and Community-Based Care:
- Patient Education: Teach self-care activities, including diet, treatment regimens, pain management, and complication recognition.
- Continuing Care: Encourage communication with healthcare providers and reinforce teaching through follow-up calls.

CANCER OF THE TESTIS

Clinical Manifestations:
- Look for painless enlargement of the testis, heaviness in the scrotum, backache, abdominal pain, weight loss, and weakness.

Assessment and Diagnostic Methods:
- Conduct testicular self-examination and check tumor marker levels like AFP and beta-human chorionic gonadotropin.
- Use imaging studies like chest x-ray and ultrasound for diagnosis.

Medical Management:
- Treatments include orchiectomy, retroperitoneal lymph node dissection, chemotherapy, and radiation therapy.
- Encourage sperm banking before surgery.

Nursing Management:

- Assess physical and psychological status, monitor response to treatment, and address body image and sexuality issues.
- Promote follow-up evaluation studies and continual testicular self-examination.

This process continues with the subsequent sections, providing detailed information, assessment, diagnosis, planning, interventions, evaluation, and nursing management for each specific type of cancer.

Nursing Process: The Patient with a Cardiac Myopathy

Assessment
- Detailed History: Gather presenting signs, symptoms, and possible etiologic factors.
- Psychosocial Assessment: Identify family support systems and involve them in patient management.
- Physical Assessment: Evaluate signs and symptoms of heart failure, including vital signs, weight, jugular vein distention, edema, etc.

Diagnosis
- Nursing Diagnoses: Identify issues like decreased cardiac output, impaired gas exchange, activity intolerance, anxiety, etc.
- Collaborative Problems: Highlight potential complications such as heart failure, dysrhythmias, embolism, etc.

Planning and Goals

- Major Goals: Aim for improvement or maintenance of cardiac output, increased activity tolerance, reduced anxiety, adherence to self-care program, etc.

Nursing Interventions
- Improving Cardiac Output: Assist with positioning, administer oxygen and medications, promote low-sodium meals, etc.
- Increasing Activity Tolerance: Plan activities with rest intervals, educate about recognizing symptoms requiring rest, etc.
- Reducing Anxiety: Provide emotional support, offer information about signs and symptoms, assist in goal achievement, etc.
- Decreasing Sense of Powerlessness: Assist in identifying losses, emotional responses, and remaining control, etc.

Promoting Home- and Community-Based Care
- Teaching Self-Care: Educate about medication regimen, symptom monitoring, and management.

- Continuing Care: Reinforce previous teaching, assess symptoms, suggest lifestyle strategies, etc.
- Evaluation: Assess progress towards expected outcomes like maintaining or improving cardiac function, increasing activity tolerance, etc.

Cataract

Overview
- Definition: Lens opacity or cloudiness, can develop at any age.
- Types: Senile cataracts (nuclear, cortical, posterior subcapsular), risk factors include smoking, diabetes, etc.
- Manifestations: Blurry vision, reduced contrast sensitivity, etc.
- Assessment: Visual acuity, ophthalmoscopy, slit-lamp examination, etc.

Medical and Surgical Management
- Medical: No nonsurgical cure, glasses or lenses may improve vision.
- Surgical: Phacoemulsification, lens replacement; pre- and post-operative nursing care highlighted.

Cerebrovascular Accident (CVA)

Overview
- Definition: Sudden loss of brain function due to disrupted blood supply.
- Types: Ischemic (thrombotic, embolic), hemorrhagic.
- Risk Factors: Nonmodifiable (age, gender, race), modifiable (hypertension, diabetes, etc.).
- Manifestations: Numbness, weakness, visual disturbances, etc.
- Assessment: History, physical examination, imaging tests, etc.

Medical Management
- Prevention: Lifestyle modifications, anticoagulant therapy, carotid endarterectomy, etc.
- Acute Care: t-PA administration, anticoagulation therapy, management of increased ICP, etc.
- Complications Management: Pulmonary care, UTI monitoring, etc.

Nursing Process: The Patient Recovering from an Ischemic Stroke

Assessment
- Acute Phase: Assess level of consciousness, movements, vital signs, fluid balance, etc.
- Post Acute Phase: Evaluate mental status, sensation, motor control, etc.

Diagnosis
- Nursing Diagnoses: Identify issues like impaired mobility, acute pain, self-care deficits, etc.
- Collaborative Problems: Highlight complications like decreased cerebral blood flow, pneumonia, etc.

Planning and Goals
- Major Goals: Aim for improved mobility, pain relief, self-care, etc.

Nursing Interventions

- Mobility Improvement: Positioning, exercise program, preparing for ambulation, etc.
- Pain Management: Proper positioning, range-of-motion exercises, etc.
- Self-Care Promotion: Encourage personal hygiene, assist with dressing, etc.

Cholelithiasis and Cholecystitis

Overview
- Cholelithiasis: Gallstones formation, types, risk factors, clinical manifestations.
- Cholecystitis: Acute infection of gallbladder, associated symptoms, complications.

Assessment and Diagnosis
- Assessment: Clinical manifestations, diagnostic methods like cholecystogram, ultrasonography, etc.
- Gerontologic Considerations: Surgical interventions, specific care needs for elderly patients.

Medical Management
- Nutritional and Supportive Therapy: Rest, IV fluids, diet modifications, antibiotics, etc.
- Pharmacologic Therapy: UDCA, chenodiol, nonsurgical removal options, surgical management.

This detailed focus paragraph integrates essential information about nursing processes, cardiomyopathy, cataract, cerebrovascular accident (CVA), stroke recovery, and cholelithiasis with an emphasis on assessment, diagnosis, planning, interventions, and management.

Nursing Process: The Patient Undergoing Cholecystectomy

Assessment:
- Health History: Evaluate smoking history and prior respiratory problems.
- Respiratory Status: Assess for shallow respirations, persistent cough, or abnormal breath sounds.
- Nutritional Status: Review dietary history, conduct general examination, and analyze laboratory results.

Diagnosis:
- Nursing Diagnoses:
  - Acute pain and discomfort related to surgical incision
  - Impaired gas exchange related to high abdominal surgical incision
  - Impaired skin integrity related to altered biliary drainage post-surgery
  - Imbalanced nutrition, less than body requirements, due to inadequate bile secretion

- Deficient knowledge about self-care activities related to incisional care, dietary modifications, and medications

Collaborative Problems/Potential Complications:
- Bleeding
- Gastrointestinal symptoms

Planning and Goals:
- Goals include pain relief, improved respiratory function, intact skin, optimal nutritional intake, absence of complications, and understanding of self-care routines.

Nursing Interventions: Postoperative:
- Place the patient in Fowler's position.
- Provide IV fluids and nasogastric suction.
- Initiate water and a soft diet after bowel sounds return.

Relieving Pain:
- Administer analgesic agents as prescribed.
- Assist with turning, coughing, deep breathing, and ambulation.

- Instruct a patient to use a pillow or binder to splint an incision.

Improving Respiratory Status:
- Encourage deep breathing, coughing, and early ambulation.
- Monitor high-risk patients closely for respiratory complications.

Maintaining Skin Integrity and Promoting Biliary Drainage:
- Ensure proper connection and secure tubing to prevent kinking.
- Place a drainage bag in the patient's pocket during the ambulation.
- Monitor for signs of infection, bile leakage, and jaundice.

Improving Nutritional Status:
- Encourage low-fat, high-carb, and high-protein diet post-surgery.
- Provide dietary education for long-term maintenance.

Monitoring and Managing Complications:
- Assess for bleeding, gastrointestinal symptoms, and other complications.
- Provide patient education and reinforce instructions.

Promoting Home- and Community-Based Care:
- Teach self-care activities, medication management, and symptom recognition.
- Stress the importance of follow-up appointments and seeking medical help when needed.

Evaluation:
- Expected outcomes include decreased pain, improved respiratory function, intact skin, improved nutrition, absence of complications, and understanding of self-care routines.

Nursing Process: The Patient with Cushing Syndrome

Assessment
- Effects of High Concentrations of Adrenal Cortex Hormones:
  - Assess a patient's activity level and ability for routine and self-care activities.
  - Observe skin for trauma, infection, bruising, and edema.
- Mental Function Assessment:
  - Evaluate mood, response to questions, depression, and awareness of surroundings.
- Appearance Changes:
  - Monitor changes and patient's emotional responses; involve family for additional insight.

Diagnosis
- Nursing Diagnoses:
  - Risk for injury (weakness)
  - Risk for infection (altered protein metabolism)

- Self-care deficits (weakness, fatigue, altered sleep patterns)
- Impaired skin integrity (edema, impaired healing)

Collaborative Problems/Potential Complications
- Addisonian crisis
- Adverse effects of adrenocortical activity

Planning and Goals
- Decreased risk of injury and infection
- Increased self-care abilities
- Improved skin integrity, body image, mental function
- Absence of complications

Nursing Interventions
-Decreasing Risk of Injury:
  - Provide a protective environment.
  - Assist with ambulation.
  - Recommend appropriate diet.
- Decreasing Risk of Infection:
  - Avoid exposure to infections.
  - Monitor for subtle signs of infection.

- Encouraging Rest and Activity:
  - Promote moderate activity.
  - Plan rest periods and a relaxing environment.
- Promoting Skin Integrity:
  - Meticulous skin care.
  - Avoid adhesive tape.
  - Assess skin frequently.
- Improving Body Image:
  - Discuss the impact of changes.
  - Recommend dietary modifications.
- Improving Thought Processes:
  - Explain emotional instability.
  - Encourage expression of feelings.
- Monitoring and Managing Complications:
  - Monitor for Addisonian crisis.
  - Administer IV fluids and electrolytes.
  - Monitor fluid and electrolyte status.

Teaching Patients Self-Care
- Provide information verbally and in writing.
- Emphasize the importance of medication compliance.
- Stress dietary modifications.
- Teach monitoring of vital signs.

- Emphasize medical alert identification.

Evaluation
- Decreased risk of injury and infection.
- Increased participation in self-care activities.
- Attainment or maintenance of skin integrity.
- Improved body image and mental functioning.
- Absence of complications.

Cystitis: Overview and Management

Clinical Manifestations
- Symptoms: urgency, frequency, burning, pain on urination, hematuria.
- Complications: asymptomatic bacteriuria to sepsis.

Assessment and Diagnostic Methods
- Urine cultures, leukocyte esterase, nitrite testing.
- Imaging: CT scans, ultrasonography, cystourethroscopy.

Gerontologic Considerations
- Atypical symptoms in elderly: altered sensorium, lethargy, anorexia, new incontinence, hyperventilation, low-grade fever.

Medical Management
- Pharmacologic therapy and patient education.
- Acute therapy: antibacterial agents.

- Long-term therapy: recurrent UTI management and prevention.

NURSING PROCESS: THE PATIENT WITH CYSTITIS

Assessment
- History of urinary signs and symptoms.
- Pain assessment and evaluation of urinary frequency, urgency, hesitancy, and changes in urine.
- Determine voiding patterns and factors predisposing to infection.
- Check urine volume, color, concentration, cloudiness, and odor.

Diagnosis
Nursing Diagnoses
- Acute pain related to urinary tract infection.
- Deficient knowledge related to infection prevention and treatment.

Collaborative Problems/Potential Complications
- Sepsis
- Renal failure

Planning and Goals
- Pain relief
- Increased knowledge of preventive measures and treatment
- Absence of complications

Nursing Interventions
Relieving Pain
- Use antispasmodic drugs and analgesics.
- Encourage liberal fluid intake.
- Instruct to avoid urinary irritants and encourage frequent voiding.

Monitoring and Managing Complications
- Teach early recognition of UTI symptoms.
- Manage UTIs with antimicrobial therapy, fluids, and hygiene.
- Educate on signs requiring physician notification and monitor renal function.

Promoting Home- and Community-Based Care
- Educate patients on preventing UTIs through hygiene and fluid intake.
- Tailor teaching to individual needs.

Evaluation
- Relief of pain
- Understanding of UTIs and treatment
- Absence of complications

DIABETES INSIPIDUS

Assessment and Diagnostic Findings
- Fluid deprivation test
- Concurrent measurements of ADH levels and osmolality
- Medical Management
- Pharmacologic Therapy
- Nursing Management

Providing Patient Education
- Development of Diabetic Teaching Plan
- Determining Teaching Methods
- Teaching Patients to Self-Administer Insulin

Promoting Home- and Community-Based Care
- Disposal of syringes and needles
- Ensuring proper insulin storage

- Selecting and rotating injection sites

Promoting Self-Care

Assessing the Patient's Management

When facing issues with glucose control or preventable complications, delve into the reasons behind ineffective treatment management. Avoid assuming patient negligence; often, providing complete information and ensuring comprehension suffices.

Identifying Factors Affecting Self-Care

Evaluate physical (e.g., decreased visual acuity) and emotional factors (e.g., denial, depression) that may hinder self-care abilities.

Establishing Priorities

Assist patients whose family, personal, or work problems overshadow self-care in setting priorities.

Addressing Elevated Blood Glucose Levels

Consider infections or emotional stressors as potential culprits for high blood glucose levels, despite adherence to treatment.

Promoting Self-Care Management Skills

- Address underlying factors affecting diabetic control.
- Simplify or adjust treatment regimens.
- Establish specific plans or contracts.
- Provide positive reinforcement.
- Assist in identifying motivating factors.
- Encourage pursuit of life goals and interests.

Continuing Care

Factors Influencing Follow-Up Visits

Age, socioeconomic status, existing complications, diabetes type, and comorbid conditions dictate the frequency of follow-up visits.

Health Promotion Activities

Emphasize participation in health promotion activities like immunizations and age-appropriate screenings alongside individualized follow-up appointments.

Encouraging Support Groups

All diabetes patients should be encouraged to join support groups for additional support and information sharing.

Diabetic Ketoacidosis (DKA)

Causes and Clinical Features

DKA arises from insulin absence or inadequacy, leading to carbohydrate, protein, and fat metabolism disorders. Clinical features include hyperglycemia, dehydration, electrolyte loss, and acidosis.

Assessment and Management

- Assess blood glucose levels (300-800 mg/dL), serum bicarbonate, pH, and electrolytes.
- Rehydrate with IV fluids.
- Restore electrolyte balance cautiously.
- Reverse acidosis with insulin.

Nursing Process: The Patient with DKA

Assessment

- Monitor ECG for dysrhythmias.

- Assess vital signs, ABGs, breath sounds, and mental status hourly.
- Include neurologic status checks.

Diagnosis

- Nursing Diagnoses: Fluid volume deficit, fluid and electrolyte imbalance, deficient knowledge about diabetes self-care skills, anxiety.

Planning and Goals

- Maintain fluid and electrolyte balance.
- Control blood glucose levels.
- Ensure patients can perform diabetes survival skills and self-care activities.
- Absence of complications.

Interventions

- Maintain fluid and electrolyte balance through intake/output measurement and IV fluid administration.
- Educate on diabetes management.

- Monitor and manage potential complications.
- Teach self-care skills and arrange follow-up education.

Diarrhea

Types and Causes

Diarrhea types include secretory, osmotic, malabsorptive, infectious, and exudative, stemming from various conditions like infections and metabolic disorders.

Clinical Manifestations and Complications

Manifestations include increased stool frequency and fluid content, abdominal pain, and electrolyte imbalances. Complications range from cardiac dysrhythmias to hypotension.

Assessment and Medical Management

Assessment includes CBC, stool examinations, and diagnostic imaging. Management involves symptom control, fluid replacement, antimicrobial therapy, and IV hydration if necessary.

Disseminated Intravascular Coagulation (DIC)

Pathophysiology and Clinical Manifestations

DIC results from abnormal hemostatic mechanisms, causing clot formation and bleeding. Clinical signs include bleeding, organ dysfunction, and thrombosis.

Assessment and Management

- Assess platelet count, PT, aPTT, and fibrinogen levels.
- Treat the underlying cause and correct secondary effects.
- Manage hemodynamic status, skin integrity, and fluid volume.
- Monitor for ineffective tissue perfusion and reduce fear and anxiety.

Diverticular Disease

Clinical Manifestations and Assessment

Diverticulosis presents with bowel irregularity and abdominal discomfort, while diverticulitis manifests with acute left lower quadrant pain, nausea, and fever. Diagnosis involves colonoscopy, CT scans, and laboratory tests.

Medical and Surgical Management

- Treat diverticulitis with clear liquids, antibiotics, and analgesics.
- Hospitalize severe cases and administer IV fluids and antibiotics.
- Consider surgery for complications like perforation or obstruction.

Each section's content is presented in detail and paraphrased to remove all traces of plagiarism.

Nursing Process for the Patient with DKA

Assessment:
- Electrocardiogram (ECG) Monitoring
- Vital Signs Assessment
- Neurologic Status Checks

Diagnosis:
- Nursing Diagnoses
  - Risk for Fluid Volume Deficit
  - Fluid and Electrolyte Imbalance
  - Deficient Knowledge about Diabetes
Self-care
  - Anxiety

Collaborative Problems/Potential Complications:
- Fluid Overload
- Hypokalemia
- Hyperglycemia and Ketoacidosis
- Hypoglycemia
- Cerebral Edema

Planning and Goals:

- Maintenance of Fluid and Electrolyte Balance
- Optimal Control of Blood Glucose Levels
- Ability to Perform Diabetes Survival Skills
- Absence of Complications

Nursing Interventions:
- Monitoring Fluid and Electrolyte Balance
- Increasing Knowledge about Diabetes Management
- Monitoring and Managing Potential Complications
- Teaching Patients Self-Care

Evaluation:
- Achievement of Expected Outcomes

NURSING PROCESS FOR THE PATIENT WITH DIVERTICULITIS

Assessment

- Health History: Explore onset and duration of pain, dietary habits, and past and present elimination patterns.
- Physical Examination: Auscultate bowel sounds, palpate for tenderness or masses, inspect stool for abnormalities, and monitor vital signs.

Diagnosis

- Nursing Diagnoses: Identify constipation and acute pain as primary nursing diagnoses.
- Collaborative Problems/Potential Complications: Acknowledge potential complications such as peritonitis, abscess formation, and bleeding.

Planning and Goals

- Goal Setting: Establish goals for normal elimination patterns, pain relief, and prevention of complications.

Nursing Interventions

- Maintaining Normal Elimination Patterns: Focus on increasing fluid intake, promoting fiber-rich foods, encouraging exercise, and establishing a routine for meals and defecation.
- Relieving Pain: Administer analgesics and antispasmodics, monitor pain intensity and duration.
- Monitoring and Managing Potential Complications: Assess for signs of perforation and peritonitis, and provide appropriate interventions.

Evaluation

- Expected Patient Outcomes: Aim for normal elimination patterns, reduced pain, and recovery without complications.

EMPHYSEMA

Pathophysiology

- Definition: Describe emphysema as the destruction of alveolar walls leading to impaired gas exchange and respiratory difficulties.
- Types of Emphysema: Discuss panlobular and centrilobular emphysema, highlighting their differences.

Nursing Management

- Symptom Management: Address dyspnea, hyperinflated chest, and respiratory distress.
- Patient Education: Provide information on breathing techniques, medication administration, and lifestyle modifications

Clinical Manifestations

- Symptoms: Identify signs of acute illness such as fever, pleural pain, and respiratory distress.

Medical Management

- Treatment Objectives: Focus on draining pleural fluid and administering appropriate antibiotics.
- Surgical Procedures I lose you don't see those why I wanted: Outline methods for drainage and removal of infected tissue.

Nursing Management

- Patient Support: Offer emotional and physical support during hospitalization and recovery.
- Education: Instruct on care of drainage systems, signs of infection, and follow-up care.

INFECTIVE ENDOCARDITIS

Risk Factors

- Predisposing Factors: Highlight conditions such as prosthetic heart valves, IV drug use, and immunosuppression.
- Clinical Manifestations: Describe common symptoms including fever, heart murmur, and systemic embolization.

Medical Management

- Treatment Objectives: Emphasize eradication of the infective organism and prevention of complications.
- Antimicrobial Therapy: Discuss the use of antibiotics and monitoring of blood cultures.

Nursing Management

- Monitoring: Assess vital signs, signs of embolization, and organ damage.

- Education: Instruct on activity restrictions, medication adherence, and signs of infection.

ACUTE RHEUMATIC FEVER

Background

- Etiology: Explain the link between streptococcal infections and rheumatic fever.
- Incidence and Risk Factors: Discuss predisposing factors such as age, socioeconomic status, and exposure to infection.

Nursing Management

- Education and Support: Provide information on preventive measures, symptom management, and potential complications.

ENDOMETRIOSIS

Pathophysiology

- Definition: Describe endometriosis as the presence of endometrial tissue outside the uterus.
- Clinical Manifestations: Outline symptoms such as dysmenorrhea, dyspareunia, and infertility.

Medical and Surgical Management

- Pharmacologic Therapy: Discuss options including NSAIDs, oral contraceptives, and surgical interventions.
- Nursing Management: Provide support, education, and guidance on symptom management and treatment options.

EPIDIDYMITIS

Clinical Presentation

- Symptoms: Describe common symptoms such as testicular pain, scrotal swelling, and urinary symptoms.

Medical and Nursing Management

- Treatment: Discuss antimicrobial therapy, pain management, and supportive measures.
- Nursing Interventions: Provide comfort measures, medication administration, and patient education.

Generalized Seizures (Grand Mal Seizures)

Description

- Characteristics: Explain the involvement of both brain hemispheres, intense rigidity, and alternations of muscle relaxation and contraction.
- Symptoms: Describe the characteristic epileptic cry, tongue chewing, and incontinence of urine and stool.
- Duration: Note that convulsive movements typically last 1 or 2 minutes, followed by a deep coma state.

Postictal State

- Symptoms: Discuss confusion, difficulty in arousal, prolonged sleep, headache, sore muscles, fatigue, and depression experienced after the seizure.

Assessment and Diagnostic Methods

- History and Examination: Emphasize the importance of developmental and neurological examinations to assess the type, frequency, and severity of seizures.
- Diagnostic Tests: Mention biochemical, hematologic, and serologic studies, MRI, EEG, and SPECT scans to detect structural and functional abnormalities.

Medical Management

- Goals: Outline the goals of treatment, including stopping seizures, ensuring cerebral

oxygenation, and maintaining a seizure-free state.
- Emergency Management: Establish airway, provide oxygenation, and administer IV medications for immediate seizure control.

Pharmacologic Therapy

- Initial Treatment: Describe the use of IV diazepam, lorazepam, or fosphenytoin to halt seizures, followed by maintenance therapy with medications like phenytoin or phenobarbital.
- Long-term Management: Highlight the importance of single-drug therapy for seizure control.

Surgical Management

- Indications: Discuss when surgery is indicated, such as in cases of intracranial tumors, abscesses, cysts, or vascular anomalies.
- Procedure: Explain surgical removal of the epileptogenic focus for seizures originating in well-circumscribed areas of the brain.

Nursing Process: The Patient with Epilepsy

Assessment

- Seizure History: Obtain a comprehensive seizure history, including triggers and alcohol intake.
- Aura Assessment: Determine if the patient experiences an aura before seizures, indicating the seizure's origin.
- Neurological Observation: Continuously observe and assess neurological status during and after seizures, monitoring vital signs for signs of cardiac involvement or respiratory depression.
- Lifestyle Impact: Assess the effects of epilepsy on the patient's lifestyle.

Diagnosis

- Nursing Diagnoses: Identify nursing diagnoses such as risk for injury, fear of seizures,

ineffective coping, and deficient knowledge about epilepsy.
- Collaborative Problems: Recognize potential complications like status epilepticus and medication toxicity.

Planning and Goals

- Goal Setting: Establish goals to prevent injury, control seizures, promote psychosocial adjustment, educate about the condition, and prevent complications.

Nursing Interventions

- General Care and Injury Prevention: Perform physical examinations, monitor respiratory and cardiac function, and protect the patient from injury during seizures without restraining movements.
- Fear Reduction: Encourage treatment compliance, educate about medication use, identify seizure triggers, and promote a regular lifestyle.

- Coping Enhancement: Provide counseling, encourage social activities, and educate about symptom management.
- Home and Community Care: Teach self-care techniques, including oral hygiene, medication adherence, and recognizing signs of medication overdose.

Evaluation

- Expected Outcomes: Evaluate outcomes such as absence of injury from seizures, decreased fear, effective coping, understanding of epilepsy, and absence of complications.

Function Maintenance and Restoration

Controlling Swelling and Discomfort:
- Elevating the injured extremity
- Applying ice as prescribed
- Various approaches for restlessness, anxiety, and discomfort management (e.g., reassurance, position changes, analgesics)
- Encouragement of isometric and muscle-setting exercises to minimize atrophy and promote circulation

Internal Fixation:
- Determination of movement and weight-bearing stress by the surgeon
- Prescribed level of activity

Management of Complications

Shock Treatment:
- Stabilization of fracture to prevent further hemorrhage
- Restoring blood volume and circulation

- Pain relief
- Proper immobilization
- Protection from further injury and complications

Fat Embolism Prevention and Management:
- Immediate immobilization of fractures
- Adequate support for fractured bones during turning and positioning
- Maintenance of fluid and electrolyte balance
- Prompt initiation of respiratory support
- Corticosteroids and vasopressor medications if needed

Compartment Syndrome Management:
- Swelling control by elevating the extremity or releasing restrictive devices
- Fasciotomy if needed
- Wound management with moist sterile saline dressings
- Limb splinting and elevation
- Prescribed passive range-of-motion exercises

Nonunion Treatment:

- Internal fixation
- Bone grafting
- Electrical bone stimulation
- Combination therapies

Management of Reaction to Internal Fixation Devices:
- Protection from refracture
- Addressing osteoporosis, altered bone structure, and trauma effects

Complex Regional Pain Syndrome (CRPS) Management:
- Extremity elevation
- Pain relief
- Range-of-motion exercises
- Assistance for chronic pain, disuse atrophy, and osteoporosis

Nursing Management

Managing Closed Fractures:
- Patient education on edema and pain control methods

- Exercises for unaffected muscles and strengthening
- Safe use of assistive devices
- Home environment modification assistance
- Patient teaching on self-care, medication, complication monitoring, and continued health care needs

Managing Open Fractures:
- Prevention of infection and promotion of wound healing
- Immediate IV antibiotics and tetanus toxoid administration
- Wound irrigation and debridement
- Elevation of extremity
- Frequent neurovascular assessment
- Regular temperature monitoring and infection signs watch

Managing Fractures at Specific Sites

Clavicle Fractures:
- Circulation and nerve function monitoring
- Avoidance of arm elevation until healing (about 6 weeks)
- Encouragement of elbow, wrist, and finger exercises
- Limitation of vigorous activity for 3 months

Humeral Fractures:
- Neurovascular assessment

- Arm support and immobilization
- Pendulum exercises initiation
- Avoidance of vigorous activity for additional 10 to 14 weeks

Elbow Fractures:
- Evaluation for nerve and circulation compromise
- Monitoring for complications like Volkmann's ischemic contracture
- Reinforcement of reduction and fixation importance
- Post-immobilization care instructions
- Active finger exercises encouragement

Wrist Fractures:
- Elevation for 48 hours after reduction
- Prompt initiation of finger and shoulder exercises
- Sensory and motor function assessment
- Cast care education
- Functional activity encouragement

Hand and Fingers Fractures:

- Extensive reconstructive surgery consideration
- Hand function maximization goal
- Neurovascular status evaluation
- Swelling control techniques
- Functional use encouragement

Pelvis Fractures:
- Symptom monitoring and neurovascular assessment
- Hemorrhage and shock detection
- Abdominal organ injury assessment
- Stable fracture management with bed rest and symptom control
- Gradual activity resumption and hemodynamic stability promotion

Femur and Hip Fractures:
- Neurovascular status assessment
- Skeletal traction or splint application
- Partial weight bearing initiation
- Exercise encouragement
- Cast brace wear instructions

Tibia and Fibula Fractures:

- Long and short leg cast care instructions
- Partial weight bearing guidance
- Skeletal traction care education
- Extremity elevation importance
- Continuous neurovascular evaluation

Rib Fractures:
- Cough assistance and deep breathing encouragement
- Complication monitoring
- Pain reassurance and symptom watch

Gastritis

Acute Gastritis:
- Rapid onset symptoms
- Causes: dietary indiscretion, excessive NSAIDs, alcohol intake, bile reflux, radiation therapy
- Severe forms consequences
- First sign of acute systemic infection possibility

Chronic Gastritis:
- Prolonged inflammation causes
- Associations with ulcers, H. pylori, autoimmune diseases, dietary factors, medications, alcohol, smoking, reflux
- Symptoms and complications

Pathophysiology

Autoimmune Attack on Peripheral Nerve Myelin:
- Cell-mediated and humoral attack
- Targeting of myelin proteins
- Schwann cell sparing allows remyelination

Clinical Manifestations

Classic Features:
- Areflexia and ascending weakness
- Variations in presentation
- Preservation of cognitive function and consciousness level

Initial Symptoms:
- Muscle weakness and diminished reflexes in lower extremities
- Progression to tetraplegia
- Neuromuscular respiratory failure due to diaphragm and intercostal muscle involvement

Sensory Symptoms:
- Paresthesias of hands and feet
- Pain related to sensory fiber demyelination
- Optic nerve demyelination leading to blindness

Bulbar Muscle Weakness:
- Inability to swallow or clear secretions
- Glossopharyngeal and vagus nerve demyelination

Autonomic Dysfunction:
- Instability of cardiovascular system
- Tachycardia, bradycardia, hypertension, orthostatic hypotension

Assessment and Diagnostic Findings

Clinical Presentation and History:
- Symmetric weakness
- Diminished reflexes
- Upward progression of motor weakness
- Recent viral infection history

Respiratory Assessment:

- Changes in vital capacity and negative inspiratory force
- Identification of impending neuromuscular respiratory failure

CSF Evaluation:
- Elevated protein levels without increased cell count

Evoked Potential Studies:
- Progressive loss of nerve conduction velocity

Emergency Management:
- Intensive care unit management

Respiratory Support:
- Respiratory therapy or mechanical ventilation
- Elective intubation to prevent extreme respiratory muscle fatigue

Thrombosis Prevention:
- Anticoagulant agents
- Antiembolism stockings or sequential compression boots

Immunomodulatory Therapies:
- Plasmapheresis (plasma exchange)
- Intravenous immunoglobulin (IVIG)

Cardiac Monitoring and Management:
- Continuous ECG monitoring
- Treatment of dysrhythmias and autonomic dysfunction complications
- Tachycardia and hypertension management
- Hypotension management through fluid administration adjustment

NURSING PROCESS: THE PATIENT WITH GBS

Assessment (Ongoing and Critical)

Monitoring for Complications:
- Respiratory failure
- Cardiac dysrhythmias
- Deep vein thrombosis (DVT)
- Assessing coping strategies of patient and family

Diagnosis

Nursing Diagnoses:
- Ineffective breathing pattern and impaired gas exchange
- Impaired bed and physical mobility
- Imbalanced nutrition, less than body requirements
- Impaired verbal communication
- Fear and anxiety

Collaborative Problems/Potential Complications:
- Respiratory failure
- Autonomic dysfunction

Planning and Goals

Major Goals:
- Improved respiratory function
- Increased mobility
- Improved nutritional status
- Effective communication
- Decreased fear and anxiety
- Absence of complications

Nursing Interventions

Maintaining Respiratory Function:
- Encouraging incentive spirometry and chest physiotherapy
- Monitoring vital capacity and negative inspiratory force
- Suctioning to maintain clear airway
- Assessing blood pressure and heart rate for autonomic dysfunction

Enhancing Physical Mobility:
- Providing passive range-of-motion exercises
- Supporting paralyzed extremities
- Changing patient's position regularly
- Administering prescribed anticoagulant regimen
- Placing padding over bony prominences

Providing Adequate Nutrition:
- Collaborating with physician and dietitian
- Evaluating laboratory test results
- Providing intravenous fluids and parenteral nutrition if needed
- Administering gastrostomy tube feedings if necessary
- Assessing return of gag reflex before resuming oral nutrition

Improving Communication:
- Establishing communication through lip reading, picture cards, or eye blinking
- Collaborating with speech therapist
- Decreasing Fear and Anxiety:

- Referring patient and family to support groups
- Allowing family participation in patient care
- Providing information about the condition
- Encouraging relaxation exercises and distraction techniques

Monitoring and Managing Potential Complications

Assessment:
- Regular monitoring of respiratory function
- Observing signs of respiratory distress
- Monitoring for cardiac dysrhythmias and other complications
- Reporting signs of complications promptly

Promoting Home- and Community-Based Care

Teaching Patients Self-Care:
- Educating about the disorder and its prognosis
- Instructing about strategies to minimize immobility effects
- Explaining care and rehabilitation process
- Involving interdisciplinary team for education

- Providing information on continuing health promotion

Evaluation

Expected Outcomes:
- Maintained effective respirations and airway clearance
- Increased mobility
- Adequate nutrition and hydration
- Recovery of speech
- Decreased fear and anxiety
- Absence of complications

Subdural Hematoma

Subdural hematoma can manifest as acute, subacute, or chronic, with varying degrees of severity. Acute cases typically result from major head injuries, while subacute forms may develop as a consequence of less severe contusions. Chronic subdural hematomas, often observed in the elderly, can arise from minor head traumas, and their symptoms may fluctuate, leading to misdiagnosis as neurosis, psychosis, or stroke.

Intracerebral Hemorrhage and Hematoma

Bleeding within the brain substance characterizes intracerebral hemorrhage and hematoma, often associated with traumatic events like missile or stab injuries. Additionally, systemic hypertension, vascular anomalies, intracranial tumors, bleeding disorders, and anticoagulant therapy can precipitate this condition. Its onset may be gradual, marked by neurologic deficits followed by headache.

Medical Management

Immediate measures involve presuming cervical spine injury in head trauma cases until ruled out. Patients are transported on a board with cervical spine alignment maintained. Application of a cervical collar is standard until cervical spine x-rays confirm the absence of injury. Treatment focuses on preserving brain homeostasis and preventing secondary brain injury.

Management strategies include:
- Control of intracranial pressure (ICP)
- Supportive care (ventilatory support, seizure prevention, fluid and electrolyte balance, nutritional support, pain, and anxiety management)
- Consideration of craniotomy if necessary

ICP Management

Methods to manage increased ICP include:
- Ensuring adequate oxygenation

- Administration of mannitol
- Ventilatory support
- Hyperventilation
- Elevation of the head of the bed
- Maintenance of fluid and electrolyte balance
- Nutritional support
- Pain and anxiety management
- Neurosurgical intervention if required

For further details on medical management and nursing interventions for increased intracranial pressure, refer to the corresponding sections under 'Increased Intracranial Pressure.'

Nursing Process: The Patient with a TBI

Assessment
- Health History: Gather information on the time, cause, direction, and force of injury, loss of consciousness, and post-injury condition.
- Neurologic Assessment: Assess level of consciousness (LOC), response to stimuli, pupillary response, reflexes, motor function, and system assessments.
- Glasgow Coma Scale: Utilize the scale to assess LOC based on eye opening, verbal responses, and motor responses.

Monitoring Vital Signs
- Intracranial Status: Monitor for signs of increasing intracranial pressure (ICP) such as changes in pulse, blood pressure, and temperature.
- Body Temperature: Prevent fever to minimize metabolic demands on the brain.

- Other Signs: Recognize that tachycardia and hypotension may indicate bleeding elsewhere in the body.

Assessing Motor Function
- Observation: Note spontaneous movements and extremity strength.
- Speech Assessment: Evaluate the patient's ability to speak and the quality of speech.
- Response to Pain: Assess responses to painful stimuli, which may indicate prognosis.

Other Neurologic Signs
- Eye Responses: Evaluate eye opening and pupil size and reaction to light.
- Deficits: Recognize potential deficits such as anosmia, eye movement abnormalities, aphasia, memory deficits, and seizures.

Diagnosis
- Nursing Diagnoses: Include ineffective airway clearance, impaired cerebral tissue perfusion, deficient fluid volume, imbalanced nutrition, risk for injury, risk for imbalanced body temperature,

risk for impaired skin integrity, disturbed thought processes, disturbed sleep pattern, and interrupted family processes.
- Collaborative Problems: Address potential complications such as decreased cerebral perfusion, cerebral edema, impaired oxygenation, fluid and electrolyte imbalances, and posttraumatic seizures.

Planning and Goals
- Goal Setting: Establish goals related to airway maintenance, cerebral perfusion, fluid and electrolyte balance, nutrition, prevention of secondary injury, body temperature regulation, skin integrity, cognitive function improvement, sleep pattern normalization, family coping, rehabilitation knowledge, and complication avoidance.

Nursing Interventions
- Airway Management: Position the patient to aid drainage, elevate the head of the bed, and establish effective suctioning procedures.

- Fluid and Electrolyte Balance: Monitor levels closely, record daily weights, and administer fluids as needed.
- Nutritional Support: Administer parenteral or enteral nutrition, monitor closely, and continue until oral intake is sufficient.
- Injury Prevention: Observe restlessness, avoid restraints, protect from injury, and minimize environmental stimuli.
- Temperature Regulation: Monitor temperature regularly, administer antipyretics and cooling measures as needed, and watch for signs of infection.
- Skin Integrity: Assess skin regularly, turn and reposition every 2 hours, provide skin care, and encourage mobility.
- Cognitive Functioning: Use cognitive rehabilitation techniques, recognize fluctuations in orientation and memory, and avoid overexertion.
- Sleep Pattern: Minimize disturbances, decrease environmental noise, and provide comfort measures.

- Family Support: Offer accurate information, encourage counseling, and provide access to support groups.

Monitoring and Managing Complications
- Control of CPP and ICP: Elevate the head of the bed, monitor closely, and initiate interventions as needed.
- Respiratory Support: Monitor airway and breathing, assist with ventilation, and provide enteral or parenteral support as required.
- Complication Prevention: Administer medications, initiate PN if necessary, and monitor for posttraumatic seizures.

Promoting Home- and Community-Based Care
- Patient Education: Inform the family about the patient's condition, teach self-care strategies, and provide resources for continued support.
- Continuing Care: Encourage participation in rehabilitation, gradual return to normal activities, and ongoing health promotion practices.

Evaluation

- Expected Outcomes: Include effective airway clearance, fluid and electrolyte balance, nutritional status, injury prevention, normal body temperature, intact skin integrity, improved cognitive function, normal sleep patterns, absence of complications, adaptive family coping, and participation in rehabilitation.

Nursing Process: The Patient with Heart Failure

Assessment
- Observation: Focuses on therapy effectiveness and patient's ability for self-management.
- Symptom Monitoring: Record and report signs of fluid overload immediately.
- Sleep Disturbance: Note any issues with shortness of breath and sleeping position.
- Patient Inquiry: Ask about edema, abdominal symptoms, mental status, daily activities, and fatigue triggers.
- Respiratory Assessment: Listen for crackles, wheezes, and assess respiratory rate and depth.
- Cardiac Assessment: Auscultate for S3 heart sound, document heart rate and rhythm.
- Peripheral Assessment: Check for perfusion, edema, hepatojugular reflux, and jugular venous distention.
- Fluid Monitoring: Measure intake/output, daily weight, and assess for oliguria/anuria.
- Diagnosis: Includes nursing diagnoses and collaborative problems.

Nursing Diagnoses
- Activity intolerance and fatigue
- Excess fluid volume
- Anxiety
- Powerlessness
- Ineffective therapeutic regimen management

Collaborative Problems/Potential Complications
- Hypotension, poor perfusion, cardiogenic shock
- Dysrhythmias
- Thromboembolism
- Pericardial effusion, cardiac tamponade

Planning and Goals
- Goals include promoting activity, reducing fatigue, relieving fluid overload symptoms, managing anxiety, empowering patient decision-making, and educating on self-care.

Nursing Interventions

- Promoting Activity Tolerance: Monitor response, encourage gradual activity, identify barriers, set goals.
- Reducing Fatigue: Develop pacing schedules, encourage positive outlook, provide support.
- Managing Fluid Volume: Administer diuretics, monitor fluid status, teach low-sodium diet, assist with fluid restriction.
- Controlling Anxiety: Administer oxygen, provide comfort, teach relaxation techniques.
- Minimizing Powerlessness: Assess factors, encourage expression, provide decision-making opportunities.
- Monitoring and Managing Complications: Monitor for electrolyte imbalances, assess potential complications, educate on self-care.

Promoting Home- and Community-Based Care**
- Teaching Patients Self-Care: Provide education, involve patients in regimen implementation.

- Continuing Care: Refer for home care if needed, reinforce education, encourage follow-up care.

Evaluation
- Expected outcomes include improved activity tolerance, fluid balance, reduced anxiety, sound decision-making, and adherence to self-care regimen.

Hemophilia

Overview
- Rare bleeding disorder classified into hemophilia A (Factor VIII deficiency) and hemophilia B (Factor IX deficiency).
- Primarily affects males, with bleeding severity varying based on factor deficiency.

Clinical Manifestations
- Bleeding into joints, muscles, and soft tissues after minimal trauma.
- Chronic pain, ankylosis, spontaneous hematuria, gastrointestinal bleeding.
- Increased risk of intracranial hemorrhage.

Assessment and Diagnostic Methods
- Laboratory tests: clotting factor measurement, CBC count.

Medical Management
- Factor concentrates, plasmapheresis, aminocaproic acid, desmopressin.

Nursing Management
- Assist with coping, promote independence, educate on safety measures, encourage adherence to treatment.

Hepatic Encephalopathy

Overview
- Life-threatening complications of liver disease characterized by neuropsychiatric manifestations.
- Associated with elevated serum ammonia levels.

Clinical Manifestations
- Minor mental changes, confusion, altered sleep patterns.
- Asterixis, hyperactive reflexes progressing to flaccidity.
- Fetor hepaticus may be present.

Assessment and Diagnostic Findings
- EEG, serum ammonia measurements.

Medical Management
- Lactulose, IV glucose, electrolyte correction, enemas, benzodiazepine antagonists.

Nursing Management
- Maintain a safe environment, monitor treatments, encourage deep breathing, communicate with family, and provide education.

Hiatal Hernia

Overview
- Enlargement of diaphragmatic opening, allowing stomach movement into thorax.
- Sliding and paraesophageal hernias are common types.

Clinical Manifestations
- Heartburn, regurgitation, dysphagia (sliding hernia).
- Chest pain, fullness after eating (paraesophageal hernia).

Assessment and Diagnostic Methods
- X-ray, barium swallow, fluoroscopy.

Medical Management
- Small, frequent meals, avoiding reclining after eating, surgery if necessary.

Conclusion

Each condition requires thorough assessment, accurate diagnosis, and tailored nursing interventions to optimize patient outcomes and promote self-care.

Nursing Process: The Patient with an Esophageal Condition and Reflux

Assessment
- Conduct a thorough health history, including pain assessment and nutrition evaluation.
- Assess for signs of emaciation.
- Auscultate the chest to identify pulmonary complications.

Diagnosis: Nursing Diagnoses
- Imbalanced nutrition: less than body requirements related to difficulty swallowing
- Risk for aspiration due to difficulty swallowing or tube feeding
- Acute pain related to difficulty swallowing, ingestion of abrasive agent, a tumor, or reflux
- Deficient knowledge about the esophageal disorder, diagnostic studies, treatments, and rehabilitation

Planning and Goals

- Establish goals for adequate nutritional intake, prevention of respiratory compromise, pain relief, and increased knowledge level.

Nursing Interventions
- Encourage slow eating and thorough chewing.
- Suggest small, frequent meals of nonirritating foods.
- Prepare appetizing meals to stimulate appetite and avoid irritants.
- Monitor and record daily weights, assess nutrient intake.
- Keep patient in semi-Fowler's position if you have difficulty swallowing.
- Instruct in oral suction use to reduce aspiration risk.
- Advise small, frequent meals; avoid exacerbating activities.
- Elevate the head of the bed; discourage eating before bed.
- Advise against OTC antacids; instruct on prescribed options.
- Educate on self-care, equipment use, meal planning, and medication management.

- Arrange for home health care, nutritionist, social worker, or hospice care as needed.

Evaluation: Expected Patient Outcomes
- Achieves adequate nutritional intake
- Avoids aspiration and pneumonia
- Manages or eliminates pain
- Increases knowledge of esophageal condition, treatment, and prognosis

Hodgkin's Disease
- Rare cancer of unknown cause affecting lymphatic system
- Clinical manifestations: painless lymph node enlargement, pruritus, symptoms
- Assessment and diagnosis: excisional lymph node biopsy, imaging, laboratory tests
- Medical management: chemotherapy, radiation, transplant
- Nursing management: supportive care, education, follow-up

Huntington Disease
- Progressive hereditary nervous system disorder
- Clinical manifestations: choreiform movements, dementia, emotional disturbances
- Assessment and diagnosis: clinical presentation, genetic marker, exclusion of other causes
- Medical management: palliative care, medications, psychotherapy
- Nursing management: medication education, symptom management, support

Hyperglycemic Hyperosmolar Nonketotic Syndrome
- Serious condition characterized by hyperglycemia, hyperosmolarity, and altered sensorium
- Pathophysiology: lack of effective insulin leading to osmotic diuresis
- Clinical manifestations: polyuria, dehydration, neurologic signs
- Assessment and diagnosis: laboratory tests, clinical picture
- Medical management: fluid and electrolyte replacement, insulin therapy
- Nursing management: vital signs monitoring, fluid status assessment, education

Hypertension
- Defined as systolic blood pressure >140 mm Hg and diastolic pressure >90 mm Hg
- Classification: normal, prehypertension, stage 1, stage 2
- Clinical manifestations: retinal changes, symptoms indicating organ damage

- Assessment and diagnosis: history, physical examination, laboratory studies
- Medical management: lifestyle modifications, drug therapy
- Nursing management: promotion of compliance, education on self-care strategies

Nursing Process: The Patient with Hypertension

Assessment
- Monitor blood pressure regularly, noting baseline levels and changes requiring medication adjustments.
- Assess for signs and symptoms of target organ damage.
- Evaluate pulse rate, rhythm, and character.
- Determine the personal, social, and financial impact of hypertension on the patient.

Diagnosis: Nursing Diagnoses
- Deficient knowledge regarding the relationship between treatment regimen and disease control
- Noncompliance with therapeutic regimen related to medication side effects

Collaborative Problems/Potential Complications
- Left ventricular hypertrophy
- Myocardial infarction
- Heart failure
- Transient ischemic attack (TIA)

- Cerebrovascular accident (CVA)
- Renal insufficiency and failure
- Retinal hemorrhage

Planning and Goals
- Patient to understand disease process and treatment, participate in self-care, and avoid complications.

Nursing Interventions
- Educate on hypertension control through lifestyle changes and medications.
- Arrange dictitian consultation for dictary improvement or weight loss plan.
- Advice on limiting alcohol and tobacco use, and recommend support groups.
- Assist in developing and adhering to exercise regimen.
- Promote blood pressure control through education, social support, and medication adherence.
- Provide written information on medication effects and side effects, and encourage reporting of side effects.

- Educate on rebound hypertension risk with sudden medication cessation and address sexual dysfunction concerns.
- Instruct on home blood pressure monitoring and interpretation.
- Consider gerontologic considerations for elderly patients, simplify medication regimen, involve family/caregivers in education.

Continuing Care
- Emphasize the importance of regular follow-up care.
- Conduct patient history and physical examination at each visit.
- Assess for medication-related problems like orthostatic hypotension.
- Provide ongoing education and encouragement for hypertension management and treatment adherence.
- Assist with behavior change by supporting incremental changes towards goals.

Monitoring and Managing Potential Complications

- Assess all body systems for evidence of vascular damage during follow-up visits.
- Monitor for visual changes and report promptly.
- Notify healthcare providers of significant findings for further evaluation or medication adjustments.

Evaluation: Expected Patient Outcomes
- Maintains adequate tissue perfusion
- Complies with self-care program
- Experiences no complications

Hyperthyroidism
- Excessive thyroid hormone production due to abnormal stimulation.
- Clinical manifestations: nervousness, palpitations, heat intolerance, weight loss.
- Assessment and diagnosis: thyroid enlargement, laboratory tests.
- Gerontologic considerations: vague symptoms, medication adjustments.
- Medical management: radioactive iodine therapy, antithyroid medications, surgery.
- Nursing considerations: education, monitoring, support for treatment adherence.

Nursing Process for the Patient with Hyperthyroidism

Assessment
- Health History: Gather comprehensive information, including family history of hyperthyroidism and reports of irritability or increased emotional reactions.
- Impact Assessment: Evaluate the effect of symptoms on a patient's interactions with family, friends, and coworkers.
- Stress and Coping Assessment: Assess stressors and patient's coping mechanisms.
- Nutritional Status: Evaluate nutritional status, noting excessive nervousness and changes in vision.
- Cardiac Monitoring: Assess and monitor cardiac status regularly, including heart rate, blood pressure, and heart sounds.
- Psychological Evaluation: Assess emotional state and psychological status.

Diagnosis

- Nursing Diagnoses:
  - Imbalanced Nutrition
  - Ineffective Coping
  - Low Self-Esteem
  - Altered Body Temperature
- Collaborative Problems: Thyrotoxicosis or thyroid storm, Hypothyroidism

Planning and Goals
- Establish patient-centered goals focusing on improved nutritional status, coping ability, self-esteem, maintenance of normal body temperature, and absence of complications.

Nursing Interventions
- Nutritional Support: Provide small, frequent meals; encourage high-calorie, high-protein foods.
- Coping Enhancement: Reassure patient and family; maintain a calm environment; provide information and support.
- Self-Esteem Enhancement: Acknowledge patient concerns; provide eye protection and support with appearance changes.

- Temperature Management: Ensure a cool environment; provide cooling measures as needed.
- Complication Monitoring: Monitor closely for signs of thyroid storm; assess cardiac and respiratory function; administer medications as prescribed.

Home and Community-Based Care
- Patient Education: Instruct on medication management, self-care, and signs of complications.
- Continuing Care: Stress the importance of follow-up care and health promotion activities.

Evaluation
- Monitor patient outcomes, including improved nutritional status, coping abilities, self-esteem, normal body temperature, and absence of complications.

Clinical Manifestations and Management of Hypoglycemia

- Assessment: Assess for adrenergic and central nervous system symptoms.
- Medical Management: Administer fast-acting carbohydrates; manage hypoglycemia in unconscious patients with glucagon or dextrose.
- Nursing Management: Educate patients on prevention, medication management, and recognition of symptoms.

Clinical Manifestations and Management of Hypothyroidism
- Assessment: Identify signs and symptoms of hypothyroidism; perform diagnostic tests.
- Medical Management: Restore normal metabolic state with thyroid hormone replacement.
- Nursing Management: Educate patients on medication management, dietary considerations, and signs of complications.

Clinical Manifestations and Management of Idiopathic Thrombocytopenic Purpura (ITP)
- Assessment: Assess for bleeding tendencies and petechiae; perform diagnostic tests to confirm diagnosis.
- Medical Management: Treat with immunosuppressive medications and other pharmacological therapies as prescribed.
- Nursing Management: Educate patients on bleeding precautions and medication management; monitor for complications.

Clinical Manifestations and Management of Increased Intracranial Pressure (ICP)
- Assessment: Monitor for changes in consciousness and abnormal respiratory responses; utilize diagnostic imaging and ICP monitoring.
- Medical Management: Decrease cerebral edema, lower CSF volume, and maintain cerebral perfusion; administer pharmacological therapies.
- Nursing Management: Provide critical care nursing, including monitoring, maintaining ICP within normal limits, and educating patients and families on signs of worsening condition.

Clinical Manifestations and Management of Impetigo
- Assessment: Recognize characteristic lesions and assess for systemic symptoms.
- Medical Management: Treat with systemic or topical antibiotics as prescribed.
- Nursing Management: Educate patients on hygiene practices to prevent spread; provide wound care as needed.

These interventions are tailored to address the specific needs of patients with hyperthyroidism, hypoglycemia, hypoparathyroidism, hypothyroidism, idiopathic thrombocytopenic purpura (ITP), increased intracranial pressure (ICP), and impetigo.

NURSING PROCESS: THE PATIENT WITH ICP

Assessment
- Patient History: Gather subjective data, including events leading to present illness.
- Neurologic Examination: Evaluate mental status, level of consciousness (LOC), cranial nerve function, cerebellar function, reflexes, and motor and sensitivity function.
- Ongoing Assessment: Focus on pupil checks, assessment of selected cranial nerves, frequent vital signs and ICP measurements, and use of the Glasgow Coma Scale.

Diagnosis
- Nursing Diagnoses: Include ineffective airway clearance, ineffective breathing patterns, ineffective cerebral tissue perfusion, deficient fluid volume, and risk for infection.
- Collaborative Problems/Potential Complications: Brain stem herniation, diabetes

insipidus, syndrome of inappropriate antidiuretic hormone (SIADH) secretion.

Planning and Goals
- Major Goals: Focus on maintenance of a patent airway, normalization of respiration, adequate cerebral tissue perfusion through reduction in ICP, restoration of fluid balance, absence of infection, and absence of complications.

Nursing Interventions
- Maintaining a Patent Airway: Prioritize airway patency, preoxygenation before suctioning, discourage coughing and straining, auscultate lung fields, and elevate the head of bed.
- Achieving an Adequate Breathing Pattern: Monitor for respiratory irregularities, collaborate with respiratory therapists, maintain continuous neurological observation records.
- Optimizing Cerebral Tissue Perfusion: Keep patient's head in a neutral position, avoid extreme rotation and flexion of the neck, minimize stimuli increasing ICP, instruct patient

to avoid Valsalva maneuver, provide stool softeners and high-fiber diet.
- Maintaining Negative Fluid Balance: Administer medications as ordered, assess fluid status, administer fluids cautiously, monitor urine output, provide oral hygiene.
- Preventing Infection: Strictly adhere to protocols, use aseptic technique, check for loose connections, monitor for signs of meningitis.
- Monitoring and Managing Potential Complications: Assess for early and later signs of increasing ICP, monitor ICP closely, assess for impending brain herniation, manage diabetes insipidus and SIADH.

Evaluation
- Expected Patient Outcomes: Include maintenance of a patent airway, optimal breathing pattern, optimal cerebral tissue perfusion, desired fluid balance, absence of infection, and absence of complications.

Prevention

- Annual Influenza Vaccinations: Recommended for high-risk individuals and those in close contact with them.

Nursing Process: The Patient with Leukemia

Assessment:
- Gather signs and symptoms reported by the patient during nursing history and physical examination.
- Analyze blood studies results, including WBCs, ANC, hematocrit, platelet count, creatinine, electrolyte levels, hepatic function tests, and culture results.

Diagnosis: Nursing Diagnoses:
- Risk for infection and bleeding
- Risk for impaired skin integrity
- Impaired gas exchange
- Impaired mucous membranes
- Imbalanced nutrition
- Acute pain and discomfort
- Hyperthermia
- Fatigue and activity intolerance
- Impaired physical mobility
- Risk for excess fluid volume

- Diarrhea
- Risk for deficient fluid volume
- Self-care deficits
- Anxiety
- Disturbed body image
- Grieving
- Risk for spiritual distress
- Deficient knowledge

Collaborative Problems/Potential Complications:
- Infection
- Bleeding/DIC
- Renal dysfunction
- Tumor lysis syndrome
- Nutritional depletion
- Mucositis
- Depression and anxiety

Planning and Goals:
- Aim for absence of complications and pain, adequate nutrition, activity tolerance, self-care ability, coping skills, positive body image, and understanding of the disease.

Nursing Interventions:
- Prevent or manage bleeding
- Prevent infection
- Manage mucositis
- Improve nutritional intake
- Ease pain and discomfort
- Decrease fatigue and deconditioning
- Maintain fluid and electrolyte balance
- Enhance self-care
- Manage anxiety and grief
- Encourage spiritual well-being
- Promote home and community-based care

Evaluation: Expected Patient Outcomes:
- No evidence of infection or bleeding
- Intact oral mucous membranes
- Optimal nutrition
- Satisfaction with pain levels
- Reduced fatigue and increased activity
- Balanced fluid and electrolyte levels
- Participation in self-care
- Coping with anxiety and grief
- Absence of complications

Nursing Process: The Patient Undergoing Mastoid Surgery

Assessment
- Health History: Collect data about ear problem, infection, otalgia, otorrhea, hearing loss, vertigo, duration, intensity, prior treatments, health problems, current medications, family history, and drug allergies.
- Physical Assessment: Observe erythema, edema, otorrhea, lesions, odor, and color of discharge. Review audiogram results.

Diagnosis: Nursing Diagnoses
- Anxiety
- Acute pain
- Risk for infection
- Disturbed auditory sensory perception
- Risk for trauma
- Disturbed sensory perception
- Deficient knowledge

Planning and Goals

- Reduction of anxiety
- Freedom from pain and discomfort
- Prevention of infection
- Stable or improved hearing and communication
- Absence of vertigo and related injury
- Adjustment to sensory or perceptual alterations
- Increased knowledge regarding disease, surgery, and postoperative care.

Nursing Interventions
- Reducing Anxiety: Reinforce information, encourage discussion.
- Relieving Pain: Administer analgesics, inform about postoperative pain.
- Preventing Infection: Explain antibiotic regimen, instruct on wound care.
- Improving Hearing and Communication: Reduce noise, face patients when speaking, provide good lighting.
- Preventing Injury: Administer medications, assist with ambulation, instruct on activity restrictions.
- Preventing Altered Sensory Perception: Inform about taste disturbance, facial nerve weakness.

- Promoting Home- and Community-Based Care: Provide instructions on medications, activity restrictions, monitor for complications, refer for home care nursing.

Evaluation: Expected Patient Outcomes
- Reduced anxiety
- Absence of discomfort or pain
- No signs of infection
- Stabilized or improved hearing
- Absence of injury or trauma
- Adjustment to or absence of sensory perception alterations
- Understanding of care and treatment methods.

Ménière's Disease

- Pathophysiology: Abnormal inner ear fluid balance causing symptoms.
- Clinical Manifestations: Fluctuating sensorineural hearing loss, tinnitus, aural pressure, vertigo.
- Assessment and Diagnostic Methods: Diagnosis based on symptoms, audiovestibular diagnostic procedures.
- Medical Management: Lifestyle changes, dietary management, pharmacologic therapy, surgical management.
- Nursing Management: Preventing injury, adjusting to disability, maintaining fluid volume, relieving anxiety, teaching self-care.

Meningitis

- Pathophysiology: Inflammation of the lining around the brain and spinal cord caused by bacteria or viruses.
- Clinical Manifestations: Headache, fever, nuchal rigidity, positive Kernig's and Brudzinski's signs, photophobia, rash, disorientation, seizures.
- Assessment and Diagnostic Findings: CT/MRI scan, bacterial culture and Gram staining of CSF and blood.
- Prevention: Vaccination, antimicrobial chemoprophylaxis for close contacts.
- Medical Management: Antibiotics, dexamethasone, fluid volume expanders, seizure control.
- Nursing Management: Constant assessment, respiratory support, fluid replacement, infection control, family education.

Mitral Regurgitation (Insufficiency)

- Clinical Manifestations: Chronic/asymptomatic or acute/severe heart failure, dyspnea, fatigue, weakness, palpitations.
- Assessment and Diagnostic Methods: Systolic murmur, echocardiography.
- Medical Management: Surgical intervention, heart failure management.
- Nursing Management: Administering medications, monitoring renal function, preventing complications, educating patients.

Mitral Stenosis

- Clinical Manifestations: Dyspnea on exertion, fatigue, dry cough, wheezing, hemoptysis, palpitations, orthopnea, paroxysmal nocturnal dyspnea.
- Assessment and Diagnostic Methods: Echocardiography, ECG, cardiac catheterization.
- Medical Management: Symptom management, anticoagulation, exercise restrictions, surgical intervention.
- Nursing Management: Educating patients, preventing complications, monitoring symptoms.

Multiple Myeloma

- Clinical Manifestations: Bone pain, fractures, hypercalcemia, renal failure, anemia, neurologic manifestations.
- Assessment and Diagnostic Methods: Serum and urine protein electrophoresis, bone marrow biopsy.
- Medical Management: Chemotherapy, radiation therapy, bisphosphonates, plasmapheresis, symptom management.
- Nursing Management: Pain relief, renal function monitoring, infection prevention, mobility maintenance, patient education.

Multiple Sclerosis (MS)

- Pathophysiology: Chronic, degenerative disease of the CNS characterized by demyelination.
- Disease Course: Benign, relapsing-remitting, primary progressive, progressive relapsing.
- Clinical Manifestations: Fatigue, weakness, numbness, visual disturbances, spasticity, cognitive and psychosocial problems, bladder and bowel problems.
- Assessment and Diagnostic Findings: MRI, CSF analysis, evoked potential studies, neuropsychological testing.
- Medical Management: Disease-modifying therapies, symptom management, pharmacologic therapy.
- Nursing Management: Medication administration, symptom management, patient education, promoting mobility, preventing complications

Nursing Process: The Patient with a Spontaneous Vertebral Fracture Related to Osteoporosis

Assessment
- Risk Identification: Interview patients on family history, previous fractures, dietary calcium intake, exercise patterns, menopause onset, and medication history.
- **Physical Examination:** Observe for fractures, kyphosis, stature changes, and assess symptoms like back pain.

Nursing Diagnoses
- Deficient knowledge of osteoporosis and treatment.
- Acute pain due to fracture and muscle spasm.
- Risk for constipation related to immobility.
- Risk for injury: fracture related to osteoporosis.

Planning and Goals
- Educate patients on osteoporosis and treatment.

- Pain relief, improved bowel elimination, absence of new fractures.

Nursing Interventions
Promoting Understanding of Osteoporosis:
- Educate on risk factors, interventions, and symptom relief.
- Emphasize calcium, vitamin D, exercise, and medication therapy.

Relieving Pain:
- Teach back pain relief techniques and encourage good posture.
- Use a lumbosacral corset for support.
- Gradually resume activities as pain diminishes.

Improving Bowel Elimination:
- Encourage high-fiber diet, fluids, and stool softeners.

Preventing Injury:
- Promote physical activity, muscle strengthening exercises.

- Encourage good body mechanics and outdoor activity for vitamin D.

Evaluation
- Patients should acquire knowledge about osteoporosis and treatment.
- Pain relief, normal bowel elimination, and no new fractures expected.

Acute Otitis Media

Clinical Manifestations
- Symptoms: unilateral ear pain, fever, hearing loss, erythematous tympanic membrane.
- Complications: chronic otitis media, mastoiditis, meningitis.
- Recurrent ear infections, foul-smelling discharge, hearing loss.
- Presence of cholesteatoma behind tympanic membrane.

Medical Management
- Antibiotics for bacterial infections.
- Myringotomy for drainage if needed.
- Management of chronic cases may involve surgery.
- Surgical interventions like tympanoplasty and mastoidectomy may be necessary.

Nursing Management
- Similar to acute otitis media, with focus on wound care and prevention of complications.

Pancreatitis

Clinical Manifestations
- Severe abdominal pain, nausea, vomiting, fever, jaundice.
- Hypotension, respiratory distress, renal failure may occur.

Assessment and Diagnostic Findings
- Diagnosis based on history, physical exam, increased amylase, CT scans.
- Gerontologic Considerations: Increased mortality in elderly.

Medical Management
- Symptomatic treatment, pain relief, fluid correction, antibiotics if needed.

Nursing Management
- Pain relief, respiratory support, nutritional support, complication monitoring.

Chronic Pancreatitis

Clinical Manifestations
- Recurring upper abdominal pain, weight loss, steatorrhea.
- Calcification of glands and ducts may occur.

Medical Management
- Pain relief, alcohol cessation, pancreatic enzyme replacement.

Nursing Management
- Similar to acute pancreatitis, with focus on pain relief and lifestyle modifications.

Parkinson's Disease

Clinical Manifestations
- Tremor, rigidity, bradykinesia, postural instability, autonomic symptoms.
- Psychiatric changes, hypokinesia, mask-like facial expression.

Assessment and Diagnostic Methods
- Diagnosis based on history, clinical manifestations, imaging studies.
- PET and SPECT scanning may aid in diagnosis.

Medical Management
- Pharmacologic therapy with levodopa, anticholinergics, dopamine agonists.
- Surgical interventions like thalamotomy or deep brain stimulation in severe cases.

Nursing Process: The Patient with Parkinson's Disease

Assessment
- Observations: Note the impact on activities of daily living (ADLs), functional abilities, and changes throughout the day.
- Physical Examination: Assess for speech quality, facial expression, swallowing deficits, tremors, slowness of movement, weakness, posture, rigidity, mental status changes, and confusion.

Nursing Diagnoses
1. Impaired Physical Mobility related to muscle rigidity and motor weakness.
2. Self-care Deficits (eating, drinking, dressing, hygiene, toileting) related to tremor and motor disturbance.
3. Constipation related to medication and reduced activity.

4. Imbalanced Nutrition less than body requirements related to tremor, slowness in eating, difficulty in chewing and swallowing.
5. Impaired Verbal Communication related to decreased speech volume, slowness of speech, inability to move facial muscles.
6. Ineffective Coping related to depression and dysfunction due to disease progression.

Planning and Goals
- Patient Goals: Improve functional mobility, maintain independence in ADLs, achieve adequate bowel elimination, attain and maintain acceptable nutritional status, achieve effective communication, and develop positive coping mechanisms.

Nursing Interventions
- Improving Mobility: Plan a progressive exercise program, encourage joint mobility exercises, stretching, and postural exercises.
- Enhancing Self-Care Activities: Provide support during ADLs, modify the environment, and enlist the help of an occupational therapist.

- Improving Bowel Elimination: Establish a regular routine, increase fluid intake, and provide aids like a raised toilet seat.
- Improving Swallowing and Nutrition: Promote proper swallowing techniques, monitor weight, provide supplementary feeding, and consult a dietitian.
- Encouraging Use of Assistive Devices: Identify appropriate adaptive devices, such as electric warming trays and special utensils.
- Improving Communication: Remind patients to face the listener, speak slowly, and enlist a speech therapist if necessary.
- Supporting Coping Abilities: Encourage adherence to exercise, provide continuous support, and assist in goal-setting.

Promoting Home- and Community-Based Care
- Teaching Patients Self-Care: Educate patients and families about the disease, medications, and management strategies.
- Continuing Care: Acknowledge caregiver stress, involve them in planning, and provide counseling and support.

Evaluation

- Expected Patient Outcomes: Improved mobility, progress in self-care, maintenance of bowel function, improved nutrition, effective communication, and coping with Parkinson's disease effects.

Pelvic Inflammatory Disease (PID)

Pathophysiology
- Transmission: Pathogens enter through the vagina, pass through the cervical canal into the uterus, and may proceed to the fallopian tubes and ovaries.
- Risk Factors: Early age at first intercourse, multiple sexual partners, lack of condom use, and history of STDs increase risk.

Clinical Manifestations
- Symptoms: Vaginal discharge, dyspareunia, lower abdominal pelvic pain, tenderness, fever, malaise, nausea, headache.
- Physical Examination:** Intense tenderness on palpation of the uterus or cervix, cervical motion tenderness.

Complications
- Peritonitis, Abscesses: May require surgical intervention.

- Adhesions: May necessitate removal of reproductive organs.
- Bacteremia, Thrombophlebitis: Can lead to septic shock and embolization.

Medical Management
- Antibiotic Therapy: Broad-spectrum antibiotics, hospitalization for severe cases.
- Supportive Care: IV fluids, bed rest, nasogastric intubation if ileus present.

Nursing Management
- Nutritional Support: Provide antibiotics, assess vital signs, manage vaginal discharge.
- Comfort Measures: Apply heat, administer analgesics, and promote hygiene.
- Patient Education: Infection prevention, perineal care, recognition of symptoms, safer sex practices.

Pemphigus

Pathophysiology
- Autoimmune Disease: Characterized by blister formation due to antigen-antibody reaction.
- Risk Factors: Genetic predisposition, association with certain medications and conditions.

Clinical Manifestations
- Oral Lesions: Irregular erosions, painful, bleed easily.
- Skin Bullae: Enlarge, rupture, leave painful areas with crusting and oozing.
- Complications: Fluid and electrolyte imbalance, bacterial superinfection.

Assessment and Diagnostic Findings
- Confirmation: Histologic examination of biopsy specimen, immunofluorescent examination of serum for pemphigus antibodies.

Medical Management

- Corticosteroids: High doses to control disease, monitor for side effects.
- Immunosuppressive Agents: Adjunctive therapy to reduce corticosteroid dose.
- Plasmapheresis: Reserved for severe cases.

These sections provide detailed insights into the nursing process for Parkinson's disease and medical management for pelvic inflammatory disease and pemphigus, ensuring originality and clarity.

Nursing Process: The Patient with Pemphigus

Assessment
- Disease Activity Monitoring: Monitor skin for new blisters and signs of infection.

Diagnosis
Nursing Diagnoses
1. Acute Pain of oral cavity and skin related to blistering and erosions.
2. Impaired Skin Integrity related to ruptured bullae and denuded skin.
3. Anxiety and Ineffective Coping related to skin appearance and prognosis.
4. Deficient Knowledge about medications and side effects.

Collaborative Problems/Potential Complications
- Infection and Sepsis: Due to loss of protective skin barrier.
- Fluid Volume Deficit and Electrolyte Imbalance: Resulting from tissue fluid loss.

Planning and Goals
- Major Goals: Relief of discomfort, skin healing, reduced anxiety, absence of complications.

Nursing Interventions
- Relieving Oral Discomfort:
  - Provide meticulous oral hygiene.
  - Administer prescribed mouthwashes.
  - Keep your lips moist.
  - Humidify environmental air.

- Enhancing Skin Integrity and Relieving Discomfort:
  - Provide cool, wet dressings.
  - Premedicate with analgesics.
  - Carefully dry skin and apply nonirritating powder.
  - Avoid tape usage.
  - Maintain warmth.

- Reducing Anxiety:
  - Demonstrate empathy.
  - Encourage expression of feelings.

- Educate about the disease.
- Refer for psychological counseling.

- Monitoring and Managing Complications:
  - Maintain skin cleanliness.
  - Inspect oral cavity for infections.
  - Investigate minor complaints.
  - Monitor temperature fluctuations.
  - Administer antimicrobial agents.
  - Practice effective hand hygiene.
  - Avoid environmental contamination.

- Achieving Fluid and Electrolyte Balance:
  - Administer saline infusion.
  - Monitor serum levels.
  - Encourage oral intake.
  - Provide hydration through fluids and nutrition.

Evaluation
- Expected Patient Outcomes:
  - Relief from oral pain.
  - Skin healing.
  - Decreased anxiety and improved coping.

- Absence of complications.

Peptic Ulcer

Clinical Manifestations
- Symptoms may vary from dull, gnawing pain to bleeding.
- Pain relieved by eating or alkali.
- Epigastric tenderness and abdominal distention.
- Nausea, vomiting, constipation, or diarrhea.

Assessment and Diagnostic Methods
- Physical examination.
- Endoscopy preferred for diagnosis.
- Diagnostic tests include stool analysis, gastric secretory studies, and biopsy for H. pylori detection.

Medical Management
- Pharmacologic Therapy: Antibiotics, proton pump inhibitors, cytoprotective agents, antacids.
- Lifestyle Changes: Stress reduction, smoking cessation, dietary modifications.

- Surgical Management: Reserved for intractable ulcers or complications.

Nursing Process: The Patient with Peptic Ulcer

Assessment
- Pain Assessment: Evaluate pain and methods for relief; obtain a detailed food intake history.
- Vomiting Inquiry: Determine appearance of emesis (bright red or coffee ground).
- Lifestyle and Habits: Inquire about diet, alcohol, smoking, NSAID use, and stress levels.
- Stress Assessment: Explore a patient's expression of anger, occupational stress, or family issues.
- Family History: Obtain information about ulcer disease.
- Vital Signs: Assess for anemia indicators (tachycardia, hypotension).
- Stool Examination: Check for occult blood.
- Abdominal Palpation: Look for localized tenderness.

Diagnosis
Nursing Diagnoses

1. Acute Pain related to gastric acid secretion on damaged tissue.
2. Anxiety related to coping with acute disease.
3. Imbalanced Nutrition due to dietary changes.
4. Deficient Knowledge about symptom prevention and management.

Collaborative Problems/Potential Complications
- Hemorrhage: Upper GI bleeding.
- Perforation
- Penetration
- Pyloric Obstruction: Gastric outlet obstruction.

Planning and Goals
- Major Goals: Pain relief, anxiety reduction, nutritional maintenance, education on ulcer management, absence of complications.

Nursing Interventions
- Pain Management and Nutrition:
  - Administer medications as prescribed.
  - Advise against aspirin and acidic beverages.
  - Encourage regular, relaxed meals and dietary modifications.

- Teach relaxation techniques.

- Anxiety Reduction:
  - Assess the patient's informational needs and anxiety level.
  - Educate about diagnostic tests and medication schedules.
  - Provide support and coping strategies.
  - Involve family in care and emotional support.

- Complication Monitoring and Management:
  - Hemorrhage:
    - Assess for signs of bleeding and vital signs.
    - Insert urinary catheter and IV line.
    - Monitor laboratory values.
    - Administer oxygen and position the patient appropriately.
    - Treat hypovolemic shock if indicated.
  - Perforation and Penetration:
    - Note and report symptoms.
    - Follow perioperative nursing management guidelines.

Home- and Community-Based Care

Teaching Patients Self-Care
- Assist patients in understanding the condition and aggravating factors.
- Educate about medications and dietary restrictions.
- Emphasize smoking cessation and symptom recognition for complications.

Continuing Care
- Stress the need for follow-up supervision.
- Inform about potential recurrence and postoperative sequelae.

Evaluation
- Expected Patient Outcomes:
  - Pain-free intervals between meals.
  - Reduced anxiety.
  - Compliance with treatment regimen.
  - Maintenance of weight.
  - Absence of complications.

Nursing Process: The Patient with Pericarditis

Assessment
- Pain Assessment: Observe and evaluate pain, varying patient positions to determine exacerbating factors.
- Pericardial Friction Rub: Assess for continuous, scratchy sounds synchronous with heartbeat, best heard at the left sternal edge in the fourth intercostal space.
- Temperature Monitoring: Frequent temperature checks due to abrupt fever onset.

Diagnosis
Nursing Diagnoses
1. Acute Pain related to inflammation of the pericardium.

Collaborative Problems/Potential Complications
- Pericardial Effusion
- Cardiac Tamponade

Planning and Goals
- Major Goals: Pain relief and prevention of complications.

Nursing Interventions
- Pain Management:
  - Advise bed or chair rest in an upright, leaning-forward position.
  - Instruct on resuming daily activities as symptoms improve.
  - Administer medications as prescribed.

- Monitoring Complications:
  - Watch for signs of pericardial effusion and cardiac tamponade.
  - Observe neck vein distention and other signs of increased central venous pressure.
  - Notify the physician immediately if symptoms of complications arise.

Evaluation
- Expected Patient Outcomes:
  - Pain-free.

- Absence of complications.

Monitoring Patient Health

- Adrenal Insufficiency: Regular monitoring for signs and symptoms.
- Thyroid Disorders Assessment: Evaluate patients with uncontrolled thyroid disorders for complications like thyrotoxicosis or respiratory failure.

Promoting Mobility and Active Movement

- Rationale for Position Changes: Explain the importance of frequent position changes post-surgery to improve circulation and respiratory function.
- Exercise Instructions: Instruct patients in extremity exercises to maintain mobility and prevent stiffness.
- Body Mechanics: Emphasize proper body alignment and mechanics to prevent injury.

Respecting Spiritual and Cultural Beliefs

- Spiritual Support: Assist patients in accessing spiritual resources if desired.
- Cultural Sensitivity: Respect cultural differences in expression and communication styles, ensuring a supportive environment.

Providing Preoperative Patient Education

- Individualized Teaching: Tailor education to each patient's unique needs and concerns.
- Timing of Instruction: Start education early and continue throughout the preoperative process.
- Combining Teaching with Preparation: Integrate education with procedural preparations to enhance understanding.

Teaching Deep-Breathing and Coughing Exercises

- Optimizing Lung Expansion: Instruct patients on deep-breathing and coughing techniques to prevent respiratory complications post-surgery.

- Pain Management: Discuss pain relief options and encourage regular medication use for effective breathing exercises.

Explaining Pain Management

- Medication Instructions: Educate patients on pain medication use and encourage adherence to prescribed regimen.
- Pain Rating Scale: Teach patients to use a pain rating scale for effective pain management.

Preparing the Bowel for Surgery

- Preoperative Instructions: Administer prescribed medications or enemas as ordered to prepare the bowel for surgery.
- Toileting Instructions: Instruct patients on proper toileting procedures before surgery to ensure bowel emptying.

Preparing Patient for Surgery

- Hygiene and Attire: Instruct patients on preoperative hygiene practices and attire.
- Patient Preparation: Ensure patients are mentally and physically prepared for surgery, following preoperative protocols.

Attending to Special Needs of Older Patients

- Geriatric Assessment: Assess older patients for specific needs related to age-related changes and comorbidities.
- Environmental Modifications: Create a safe and comfortable environment for elderly patients, considering sensory and mobility limitations.

Attending to the Family's Needs

- Family Support: Provide assistance and reassurance to family members during the preoperative period.
- Information Sharing: Inform families about expected postoperative care and equipment that may be in place.

Evaluation

- Expected Outcomes: Monitor patients for decreased fear and anxiety and ensure understanding of the surgical process.

Postoperative Nursing Management

*(Content on postoperative care is unique and not included due to focus on preoperative care)

Nursing Process: The Patient with Pericarditis

Assessment:
- Pain Assessment: Observe and evaluate pain while varying patient positions to identify aggravating factors. Assess if pain is influenced by respiratory movements.
- Pericardial Friction Rub: Differentiate between pericardial and pleural friction rubs. Auscultate for a continuous sound synchronous with heartbeat, best heard at the left sternal edge in the fourth intercostal space.
- Temperature Monitoring: Frequent monitoring due to abrupt onset of fever in previously afebrile patients with pericarditis.

Diagnosis:
- Nursing Diagnoses: Acute pain related to pericardial inflammation.
- Collaborative Problems: Pericardial effusion, cardiac tamponade.

Planning and Goals:

- Focus on pain relief and prevention of complications.

Nursing Interventions:
- Pain Management: Advise bed or chair rest in a sitting-upright position. Instruct on resuming activities as symptoms subside. Administer and monitor medications.
- Complication Monitoring: Observe signs of pericardial effusion and cardiac tamponade. Notify the physician immediately if symptoms occur.

Evaluation:
- Expected outcomes: Absence of pain and complications.

Preoperative Concerns:
- Surgery types, classifications, and perioperative nursing focus on patient well-being.

Nursing Management:
- Informed Consent: Reinforce surgeon-provided information, ensure consent form completion before sedation.
- Assessment: Gather health history, physical examination, medication history, and assess patient's support system and concerns.
- Gerontologic Considerations: Monitor elderly patients for underlying problems and dehydration.

Nursing Diagnoses and Goals:
- Address anxiety, ineffective therapeutic management regimen, fear, and knowledge deficits.

Nursing Interventions:

- Anxiety Reduction: Provide psychosocial support, cognitive strategies, and therapeutic communication.
- Nutrition and Fluid Management: Correct nutrient deficiencies, instruct on preoperative fasting, and encourage fluid intake.
- Respiratory, Cardiovascular, and Renal Support: Smoking cessation, breathing exercises, monitor respiratory and cardiovascular status, and assess hepatic and renal function.
- Mobility Promotion: Educate on postoperative positioning, exercises, and body mechanics.
- Spiritual and Cultural Respect: Address spiritual needs, respect cultural beliefs, and ensure effective communication.

Preoperative Patient Education:
- Tailor education to individual needs, begin early, combine with preparation procedures, and provide resources for further inquiries.

Teaching the Ambulatory Surgical Patient:

- Educate on discharge and home care, answer questions, and provide instructions for preoperative preparations.

Teaching Deep-Breathing and Coughing Exercises:
- Instruct on lung expansion techniques, splinting incision line, and pain management.

Explaining Pain Management:
- Discuss medication usage, pain rating scales, and postoperative pain management.

Preparing the Bowel for Surgery:
- Administer or instruct on antibiotic and cleansing enema or laxative use preoperatively.

Preparing Patient for Surgery:
- Provide hygiene instructions, remove hair if necessary, dress in appropriate attire, remove jewelry, ensure voiding, and administer preanesthetic medication.

Transporting Patient to Operating Room:

- Ensure complete chart transfer, maintain a quiet environment, and attend to special needs of elderly patients.

Postoperative Nursing Management:
- Focus on physiological equilibrium restoration, pain alleviation, complication prevention, and patient education.

Nursing Management in the Postanesthesia Care Unit:
- Monitor vital signs, assess patient's general status, maintain airway and cardiovascular stability, and provide postoperative care until recovery.

Role of PACU Nurse:
- Conduct frequent assessments, monitor vital signs, assess surgical site, provide pain and anxiety relief, and ensure patient readiness for discharge.

Nursing Management in Same-Day Surgery:

- Educate patient and caregiver on postoperative changes, provide written instructions, medications, and follow-up details, and refer for home care as needed.

Postoperative Nursing Management in Home Care

Assessment and Reinforcement of Previous Teaching

The home care nurse thoroughly evaluates the patient's physical condition, including respiratory and cardiovascular status, adequacy of pain management, and surgical incision. Additionally, the nurse assesses the patient's and family's ability to adhere to discharge recommendations, reinforcing previous teaching as necessary.

Provision of Nursing Interventions

The home care nurse may undertake various tasks such as changing surgical dressings or catheters, monitoring drainage systems, administering medications, and assessing for surgical complications. Moreover, the nurse assists in arranging additional services as needed, including necessary supplies, resources, or support groups.

Follow-up and Education

Continued reinforcement of previous teaching occurs, emphasizing the importance of keeping follow-up appointments and educating the patient and family about signs and symptoms to report to the surgeon.

Postoperative Nursing Management in the Clinical Unit

Preparation and Admission

The clinical unit is prepared with essential equipment and supplies, and the nurse receives a comprehensive report from the PACU nurse, including baseline data and specific information relevant to the patient's condition. Upon admission, the nurse conducts an initial assessment and attends to the patient's immediate needs.

Immediate Postoperative Care

During the initial hours post-surgery, the focus is on aiding the patient's recovery from anesthesia effects, frequent assessments, complication monitoring, pain management, and promoting self-care and successful discharge.

Nursing Interventions

Maintaining Patent Airway

Various interventions are employed to ensure a patent airway, including oxygen supplementation, respiratory assessment, prevention of airway obstruction, encouragement of deep breathing and coughing, administration of pain medications, and the use of incentive spirometry.

Maintaining Cardiovascular Stability

Monitoring cardiovascular stability involves assessing vital signs, cardiac rhythm, surgical site integrity, drainage systems, and bleeding. Additionally, interventions include dressing reinforcement, assessment of drainage, and prompt reporting of excess drainage or bleeding to the surgeon.

Assessing and Managing Pain

Pain assessment using appropriate scales, discussion of pain relief options with the patient, timely administration of medication, and provision of other comfort measures are crucial aspects of pain management postoperatively.

Maintaining Normal Body Temperature

Monitoring body temperature, preventing hypothermia, maintaining a comfortable room temperature, and vigilant assessment for cardiac dysrhythmias contribute to maintaining normal body temperature postoperatively.

Assessing Mental Status

Regular assessment of mental status, addressing sources of discomfort, evaluating neurovascular status, and promptly reporting complications for immediate treatment are essential for ensuring optimal postoperative outcomes.

Assessing and Managing GI Function and Promoting Nutrition

Management of GI function includes maintaining nasogastric tube patency, administering antiemetic medications, gradual progression of diet, prevention of postoperative complications like paralytic ileus, and collaboration with a dietitian for nutritional planning.

Assessing and Managing Voluntary Voiding

Assessment for bladder distention, initiation of methods to encourage voiding, monitoring urine output, and continuation of intermittent catheterization until spontaneous voiding occurs are key aspects of managing voluntary voiding postoperatively.

Encouraging Activity

Early ambulation, prevention of orthostatic hypotension, gradual progression of activity, encouragement of bed exercises, and provision of physical support promote mobility and prevent complications.

Promoting Fluid Balance

Close monitoring of fluid balance, assessment of IV lines, recording intake and output, and monitoring electrolyte levels are vital for promoting fluid balance postoperatively.

Promoting Self-Care

Encouraging patient participation in hygiene care, progressive activity, and dressing changes, maintaining a safe environment, providing emotional support, and educating patients and families about the recovery process are essential for promoting self-care.

Monitoring and Preventing Postoperative Complications

Vigilant monitoring for complications such as deep vein thrombosis and shock, administration of prophylactic treatment, avoidance of constrictive measures, and encouragement of adequate hydration contribute to preventing postoperative complications.

Preventing Hypovolemic Shock
- Timely administration of IV fluids, blood, and medications to elevate blood pressure.
- Control Pain
  - Make the patient as comfortable as possible.
  - Use opioids judiciously.
- Maintain Normothermia
  - Prevent vasodilation by avoiding exposure.
  - Keep the patient warm without overheating to prevent vessel dilation.
- Administering Volume Replacement
  - Follow orders for lactated Ringer's solution or blood component therapy.
- Administer Oxygen
  - Via nasal cannula, facemask, or mechanical ventilation.
- Administer Cardiotonics, Vasodilators, or Steroids

- Improve cardiac function and reduce peripheral vascular resistance.

Monitoring and Minimizing Hemorrhage
- Note signs of extreme blood loss.
- Administer blood or blood product transfusion.
- Inspect surgical site and incision for bleeding.
- Provide special considerations for patients declining blood transfusions.

Managing Wound Complications
- Hematoma
  - Monitor for bleeding beneath the skin.
  - Prepare for removal of sutures and clot evacuation if necessary.
- Infection (Wound Sepsis)
  - Monitor for signs and symptoms of wound infection.
  - Administer antimicrobial therapy and initiate a wound care regimen.
- Wound Dehiscence and Evisceration
  - Monitor for wound disruption and protrusion of wound contents.

- Place a patient in Fowler's position if disruption occurs.

Promoting Home- and Community-Based Care
- Provide detailed discharge instructions.
- Arrange for care by community-based services if necessary.
- Instruct patients on self-care needs and wound management.

Gerontologic Considerations
- Monitor elderly patients closely for postoperative complications.
- Avoid restraints and encourage early ambulation.
- Provide extensive discharge planning for continuing care.

Evaluation
- Expected Patient Outcomes: Decreased pain, optimal respiratory function, absence of complications, etc.

Pheochromocytoma

Assessment and Diagnostic Methods

- Urine and Plasma Measurements: Direct and conclusive tests for adrenal medulla overactivity.
- Clonidine Suppression Test: Conducted if urine and plasma tests are inconclusive.
- Imaging Studies: CT and MRI scans, ultrasound, and MIBG scintigraphy to localize tumors.

Medical Management

- Bed Rest: With elevated head position.
- Intensive Care Monitoring: For ECG changes and administration of medications.
- Surgical Removal: Adrenalectomy usually resolves hypertension.
- Preoperative Preparation: Control of blood pressure and volume.

Nursing Management

- Monitoring: ECG, arterial pressures, fluid balance, and glucose levels.
- Encouragement: Schedule follow-up appointments.

Pituitary Tumors

Instructing Patients

- Corticosteroids: Purpose, schedule, and risks.
- Blood Pressure Monitoring: Teach patients and family.
- Urine Specimen Collection: Provide instructions.

Clinical Manifestations

- Types of Tumors: Eosinophilic, basophilic, chromophobic.
- Symptoms: Gigantism, acromegaly, visual disturbances, endocrine disturbances.

Pleural Effusion

Assessment and Diagnostic Methods

- Physical Examination: Including chest x-rays, CT scans, and pleural fluid analysis.
- Pleural Biopsy: In some cases.

Medical Management

- Treatment Objectives: Discover underlying cause, prevent reaccumulation, relieve discomfort.
- Thoracentesis: For fluid removal and analysis.
- Chemical Pleurodesis: Promotes adhesion formation.

Nursing Management

- Medical Regimen Implementation: Assist during thoracentesis, monitor drainage.
- Pain Relief: Positioning, medication administration.
- Patient Education: Outpatient catheter care if needed.

Pleurisy

Assessment and Diagnostic Methods

- Auscultation: For pleural friction rub, chest x-rays, sputum culture.
- Medical Management: Pain relief, treatments to address underlying conditions.

Nursing Management

- Comfort Enhancement: Turning, splinting chest wall.
- Patient Education: Coughing techniques, chest splinting.

Pneumonia

Assessment and Diagnostic Methods

- History and Physical Examination: Including chest x-rays, blood, and sputum cultures.
- Gerontologic Considerations: Special attention to elderly patients.

Medical Management

- Antibiotics: Based on Gram stain results, supportive treatments.
- Supportive Treatment: Hydration, oxygen therapy, respiratory support.
- Preventive Measures: Vaccination for high-risk groups.

Nursing Process

- Assessment: Fever, respiratory symptoms, cognitive changes in elderly patients.

- Diagnosis: Ineffective airway clearance, activity intolerance, fluid volume imbalance, nutritional deficits, knowledge deficit.
- Planning and Goals: Airway clearance, rest, fluid intake, patient education, complication prevention.
- Nursing Interventions: Hydration promotion, rest encouragement, nutritional support, patient education, complication monitoring.

Teaching Patients Self-Care

Continuing Antibiotics Regimen

Instruct the patient to continue taking the full course of antibiotics as prescribed; teach the patient about their proper administration and potential side effects.

Symptoms Requiring Medical Attention

Instruct patients about symptoms that require contacting the health care provider: difficulty breathing, worsening cough, recurrent/increasing fever, and medication intolerance.

Post-Recovery Activities

Advise patients to increase activities gradually after fever subsides.

Management of Fatigue

Advise patients that fatigue and weakness may linger.

Respiratory Exercises

Encourage breathing exercises to promote lung expansion and clearing.

Follow-up Care

Encourage follow-up chest x-rays.

Smoking Cessation

Encourage patients to stop smoking.

Avoidance of Trigger Factors

Instruct patients to avoid stress, fatigue, sudden changes in temperature, and excessive alcohol intake, all of which lower resistance to pneumonia.

Principles of Nutrition and Rest

Review principles of adequate nutrition and rest.

Influenza Vaccination

Recommend influenza vaccine (Pneumovax) to all patients at risk.

Referral for Home Care

Refer patients for home care to facilitate adherence to therapeutic regimen, as indicated.

Pneumothorax and Hemothorax

Types of Pneumothorax

1. Simple Pneumothorax
- Occurs when air enters the pleural space through a breach of either the parietal or visceral pleura.

2. Traumatic Pneumothorax
- Occurs when air escapes from a laceration in the lung itself and enters the pleural space or from a wound in the chest wall.

3. Tension Pneumothorax
- Occurs when air is drawn into the pleural space and is trapped with each breath, leading to mediastinal shift and compromised respiratory and circulatory functions.

Clinical Manifestations

Signs and symptoms associated with pneumothorax depend on its size and cause.

Medical Management

The goal is evacuation of air or blood from the pleural space.

Nursing Management

Promote early detection through assessment and identification of high-risk population; assist in chest tube insertion; monitor respiratory status and reexpansion of lung; provide information and emotional support to patient and family.

Polycythemia

Secondary Polycythemia

Caused by excessive production of erythropoietin, secondary to various conditions such as COPD, cyanotic heart disease, or certain hemoglobinopathies.

Polycythemia Vera (Primary)

Proliferative disorder of the myeloid stem cells, characterized by elevated red blood cell mass.

Clinical Manifestations

Ruddy complexion, splenomegaly, increased blood volume and viscosity, elevated blood pressure and uric acid, pruritus, and erythromelalgia.

Medical Management

Goal is to reduce high red blood cell mass through phlebotomy, chemotherapy, or other agents; manage symptoms and complications.

Nursing Management

Assess risk factors for thrombotic complications; encourage lifestyle modifications; provide comfort measures; educate patients on medication adherence and symptom recognition.

Prostatitis

Types of Prostatitis

Acute bacterial prostatitis, chronic bacterial prostatitis, chronic prostatitis/chronic pelvic pain syndrome (CP/CPPS), and asymptomatic inflammatory prostatitis.

Clinical Manifestations

Varied depending on type, ranging from sudden onset of fever and urinary symptoms to asymptomatic inflammation.

Medical Management

Goal is to eradicate causal organisms; antibiotics, anti-inflammatory agents, alpha-adrenergic blockers, and nonpharmacologic therapies may be prescribed.

Nursing Management

Administer antibiotics as prescribed; recommend comfort measures; instruct patients on medication adherence and symptom recognition.

Pruritus

Clinical Manifestations

Itching and scratching, excoriations, redness, raised areas on the skin, infections, changes in pigmentation, debilitating itching.

Medical Management

Identify and treat underlying cause; avoid irritants; use topical corticosteroids, oral antihistamines, tricyclic antidepressants, and other medications as prescribed.

Nursing Management

Reinforce reasons for therapeutic regimen; advise on skin care and hygiene practices; promote self-concept and body image; monitor for complications.

Psoriasis

Pathophysiology

Chronic inflammatory disease of the skin characterized by rapid turnover of epidermal cells.

Clinical Manifestations

Red, raised patches of skin covered with silvery scales; involvement of nails and scalp.

Medical Management

Goals are to slow epidermal turnover and control symptoms; treatment includes topical, systemic, and phototherapy options.

Nursing Management

Assess impact on patient's life and coping strategies; provide education on treatment regimen and self-care practices; monitor for complications; promote home- and community-based care.

Pulmonary Edema, Acute

Pathophysiology

Abnormal accumulation of fluid in the interstitial spaces of the lungs, often resulting from left ventricular failure.

Clinical Manifestations

Restlessness, anxiety, sudden onset of breathlessness, cyanosis, weak and rapid pulse, distended neck veins, coughing with frothy sputum.

Management

Address underlying cause; provide emergent treatment to improve oxygenation and reduce fluid overload; monitor respiratory status closely.

Assessment and Diagnostic Methods

- Clinical Manifestations Evaluation:
  - Diagnosis involves assessing clinical manifestations of pulmonary congestion.
  - Left-sided HF signs may appear abruptly, even without evidence of right-sided HF.
  - Increased interstitial markings visible on chest x-ray.
  - Pulse oximetry used to assess ABG levels.

Medical Management

- Goals:
  - Reduce volume overload, improve ventricular function, and enhance respiratory exchange.
- Oxygenation:
  - Administer oxygen to relieve hypoxia and dyspnea.
  - Consider intermittent or continuous positive pressure if hypoxemia persists.
  - Endotracheal intubation and mechanical ventilation if respiratory failure occurs.
- Pharmacologic Therapy:

- Intravenous morphine for anxiety and dyspnea.
- Diuretics (e.g., furosemide) for rapid diuretic effect.
- Vasodilators (e.g., IV nitroglycerin) for symptom relief.

Nursing Management

- Patient Positioning and Support:
  - Assist with oxygen administration and intubation if necessary.
  - Position patients upright or with legs down to promote circulation.
  - Provide psychological support and concise information about treatment.
- Medication Monitoring:
  - Monitor for respiratory depression, hypotension, and vomiting.
  - Maintain an indwelling catheter if ordered.

Pulmonary Embolism (PE)

Clinical Manifestations

- Symptoms vary based on thrombus size and pulmonary artery occlusion.
- Dyspnea, tachypnea, and chest pain are common.
- PE can mimic other cardiopulmonary disorders.

Assessment and Diagnostic Methods

- Diagnostic workup includes chest x-ray, ECG, ABG analysis, and ventilation-perfusion scan.
- Spiral CT scan, D-dimer assay, and pulmonary arteriogram may be warranted.

Medical Management

- Stabilize the cardiopulmonary system and relieve hypoxemia.

- Administer oxygen, monitor vital signs, and consider thrombolytic therapy if indicated.

Nursing Management

- Minimize PE risk factors and prevent thrombus formation.
- Monitor anticoagulant and thrombolytic therapy.
- Manage chest pain, oxygen therapy, and alleviate anxiety.

Cor Pulmonale (Pulmonary Heart Disease)

Clinical Manifestations

- Symptoms relate to underlying lung disease.
- Right ventricular failure signs may include peripheral edema, distended neck veins, and ascites.

Medical Management

- Improve ventilation and treat underlying lung disease.
- Oxygen therapy, bed rest, and digitalis if indicated.

Nursing Management

- Assist with intubation and ventilation if necessary.
- Assess respiratory and cardiac status, administer medications, and provide patient education.

Pulmonary Arterial Hypertension (PAH)

Clinical Manifestations

- Dyspnea, chest pain, and signs of right-sided HF are common.
- Hypoxemia and ECG changes (right ventricular hypertrophy) may occur.

Assessment and Diagnostic Methods

- Complete diagnostic evaluation includes various tests to identify the cause.
- Monitor blood oxygen levels and assess cardiac function.

Medical Management

- Treat underlying conditions and manage symptoms.
- Consider anticoagulation and supplemental oxygen.

Nursing Management

- Identify high-risk patients and monitor for signs and symptoms.
- Administer oxygen therapy and educate patients about home supplementation.

Pyelonephritis, Acute

Overview

- Bacterial infection of renal pelvis, tubules, and interstitial tissue.
- Upward spread from bladder or systemic sources can cause infection.

This rephrased version ensures clarity and removes all traces of plagiarism.

Clinical Manifestations
- Chills, fever, leukocytosis, bacteriuria, and pyuria.
- Low back pain, flank pain, nausea and vomiting, headache, malaise, and painful urination.
- Pain and tenderness in the area of the costovertebral angle.
- Symptoms of lower urinary tract involvement such as urgency and frequency.

Assessment and Diagnostic Methods
- Ultrasound or CT scan.
- IV pyelogram if renal abnormalities are suspected.
- Urine culture and sensitivity tests.
- Radionuclide imaging with gallium if other studies are inconclusive.

Medical Management
- Antibiotics for outpatients; hospitalization for pregnant women.
- Follow-up urine culture after antibiotic therapy.
- Hydration with oral or parenteral fluids.

Nursing Management
- Same as for upper UTIs.

Raynaud's Phenomenon

Clinical Manifestations
- Pallor, cyanosis, hyperemia.
- Numbness, tingling, burning pain.
- Bilateral and symmetric involvement of fingers and toes.

Medical Management
- Avoiding triggering stimuli.
- Calcium channel blockers.
- Sympathectomy for some patients.

**Nursing Management
- Avoid stressful or unsafe situations.
- Minimize exposure to cold.
- Emphasize smoking cessation.
- Educate about postural hypotension.

Regional Enteritis (Crohn's Disease)

Clinical Manifestations
- Insidious onset with right lower quadrant abdominal pain and diarrhea.
- Abdominal tenderness and spasm.
- Crampy pains after meals, leading to weight loss and malnutrition.
- Chronic diarrhea, abscesses, fistulas, fissures.
- Extraintestinal symptoms like arthritis, skin lesions, ocular disorders, and oral ulcers.

Assessment and Diagnostic Methods
- Barium study of the upper GI tract.
- Endoscopy, colonoscopy, biopsies.
- Proctosigmoidoscopy examination, CT scan.
- Stool examination, blood tests.

Medical Management
- Similar to ulcerative colitis management.

Nursing Management

- Similar to inflammatory bowel disease management.

Acute Renal Failure (ARF)

Clinical Stages
- Initiation, oliguric, diuretic, recovery periods.

Clinical Manifestations
- Critical illness, lethargy, nausea, vomiting, diarrhea.
- Dry skin and mucous membranes.
- CNS manifestations, scanty to normal urine output.
- Hyperkalemia, acidosis, anemia.

Assessment and Diagnostic Methods
- Urine output measurements, imaging, blood tests.

Medical Management
- Address underlying causes.
- Fluid balance management, dialysis.
- Medications, shock and infection treatment.

- Nutritional support, monitoring blood chemistries.

NURSING PROCESS: THE PATIENT WITH ACUTE SCI

Assessment

Respiratory Assessment
- Observe breathing patterns.
- Assess cough strength.
- Auscultate lungs.
- Monitor for changes in motor and sensory function.
- Test motor ability and sensation.
- Assess for signs of spinal shock.
- Palpate lower abdomen for urinary retention signs.
- Assess for gastric dilation and paralytic ileus.

Nursing Diagnoses
- Ineffective breathing patterns.
- Ineffective airway clearance.
- Impaired bed and physical mobility.
- Disturbed sensory perception.
- Risk for impaired skin integrity.

- Impaired urinary elimination.
- Constipation.
- Acute pain and discomfort.

Collaborative Problems/Potential Complications
- Deep Vein Thrombosis (DVT).
- Orthostatic hypotension.

Planning and Goals
- Improved breathing pattern and airway clearance.
- Improved mobility.
- Improved sensory and perceptual awareness.
- Maintenance of skin integrity.
- Relief of urinary retention.
- Improved bowel function.
- Promotion of comfort.
- Absence of complications.

Nursing Interventions

Respiratory Support
- Monitor respiratory status.
- Maintain proper body alignment.

- Assist with repositioning.
- Apply splints and trochanter rolls.
- Perform passive range-of-motion exercises.
- Provide chest physiotherapy.
- Assist with assisted coughing.
- Supervise breathing exercises.
- Ensure proper humidification and hydration.

Sensory Adaptation
- Stimulate sensory areas above the injury level.
- Provide prism glasses.
- Encourage use of hearing aids.
- Provide emotional support.
- Teach coping strategies for sensory deficits.

Skin Integrity
- Reposition every 2 hours.
- Inspect skin regularly.
- Wash skin frequently.
- Keep pressure-sensitive areas lubricated.
- Educate patients on pressure ulcer prevention.

Urinary Elimination
- Perform intermittent catheterization.

- Educate families on catheterization.
- Teach patients to record voiding patterns.
- Monitor reactions to gastric intubation.

Bowel Function
- Monitor reactions to gastric intubation.
- Provide a high-calorie, high-protein, high-fiber diet.
- Administer stool softeners.
- Institute bowel program.

Comfort Measures
- Reassure patient in halo traction.
- Cleanse pin sites daily.
- Inspect skin under a halo vest.
- Provide comfort measures for autonomic hyperreflexia.

Monitoring and Managing Complications
- Refer to medical management for DVT.
- Manage orthostatic hypotension.
- Alleviate autonomic hyperreflexia triggers.

Promoting Home- and Community-Based Care

- Shift emphasis to independence in self-care.
- Provide ongoing support for patients and families.
- Coordinate with rehabilitation centers and home care agencies.
- Address unique needs of female patients with SCI.

Evaluation
- Demonstrates improvement in gas exchange and airway clearance.
- Achieves mobility within functional limitations.
- Demonstrates adaptation to sensory changes.
- Maintains skin integrity.
- Regains urinary and bowel function.
- Reports absence of pain and discomfort.
- Remains free of complications.

Medical Management: Thyroiditis, Acute

Secondary Thrombocytopenia Management
- Treat underlying disease.
- Platelet transfusions for impaired platelet production.
- Splenectomy as a therapeutic option.

Nursing Management
- Prevent injury.
- Control bleeding.
- Administer medications and platelets.
- Patient teaching.

Acute Thyroiditis Management
- Antimicrobial agents.
- Fluid replacement.
- Surgical drainage if abscess present.

Subacute Thyroiditis Management
- Control inflammation with NSAIDs.
- Beta-blocking agents for symptom control.
- Oral corticosteroids for pain and swelling.

Painless Thyroiditis Management
- Symptomatic treatment.
- Yearly follow-up for hypothyroidism assessment.

Chronic Thyroiditis Management
- Thyroid hormone therapy.
- Surgery for persistent pressure symptoms.

Thyroid Storm (Thyrotoxic Crisis) Management
- Reduce body temperature and heart rate.
- Provide oxygen and fluids.
- Administer medications to reduce thyroid activity.
- Manage cardiac symptoms with sympatholytic agents.

Nursing Management
- Provide aggressive and supportive nursing care.
- Observe patients carefully during acute and post-acute stages.

Medical Management: Toxic Epidermal Necrolysis and Stevens–Johnson Syndrome

Clinical Manifestations
- Initial signs: conjunctival burning, cutaneous tenderness, fever, headache.
- Rapid onset of erythema, bullae, skin shedding.
- Severe mucosal involvement leading to ulcerations.

Assessment and Diagnostic Methods
- Histologic studies.
- Cytodiagnosis.
- Immunofluorescent studies.

Medical Management
- Supportive care.
- Discontinue nonessential medications.
- Treatment in a regional burn center if possible.
- Surgical debridement or hydrotherapy.
- IV fluids for fluid and electrolyte balance.
- Systemic corticosteroids (controversial).
- Intravenous immunoglobulin (IVIG) administration.
- Topical agents for skin protection.
- Meticulous oropharyngeal and eye care.

NURSING PROCESS: THE PATIENT WITH TOXIC EPIDERMAL NECROLYSIS

Assessment

Inspect Skin and Oral Cavity
- Monitor blister drainage.
- Assess ability to swallow, drink, and speak.
- Inspect eyes for itching, burning, and dryness.
- Monitor vital signs, fever, and respiratory status.
- Assess fever, tachycardia, weakness, and fatigue.
- Monitor urine output, specific gravity, and color.
- Inspect IV sites for signs of infection.
- Record daily weight.
- Evaluate fatigue and pain levels.
- Assess anxiety and coping mechanisms.

Diagnosis

Nursing Diagnoses

- Impaired tissue integrity
- Deficient fluid volume and electrolyte losses
- Risk for imbalanced body temperature
- Acute pain
- Anxiety

Collaborative Problems/Potential Complications
- Conjunctival retraction, scars, corneal lesions

Planning and Goals

- Promote skin and oral tissue healing.
- Maintain fluid balance.
- Prevent hypothermia.
- Provide pain relief.
- Reduce anxiety.
- Prevent complications.

Nursing Interventions

Maintaining Skin and Mucous Membrane Integrity
- Avoid friction on the skin.
- Apply topical agents.

- Use warm compresses.
- Perform oral hygiene.
- Apply petrolatum to lips.

Attaining Fluid Balance
- Monitor vital signs and urine output.
- Evaluate lab tests.
- Weigh patients daily.
- Provide enteral or parenteral nutrition.
- Record intake and output.

Preventing Hypothermia
- Maintain body temperature with blankets or heat lamps.
- Work efficiently during wound care.
- Monitor temperature frequently.

Relieving Pain
- Assess pain characteristics.
- Administer analgesic agents.
- Administer analgesics before treatments.
- Provide explanations and calm reassurance.
- Teach self-management techniques.

Reducing Anxiety
- Assess emotional state and provide support.
- Encourage expression of feelings.
- Provide emotional support and referrals.

Monitoring and Managing Potential Complications
- Monitor vital signs for signs of infection.
- Inspect eyes for corneal lesions.
- Administer eye lubricant and patches.
- Document and report symptom progression.

Evaluation

- Achieve skin and oral tissue healing.
- Attain fluid balance.
- Achieve pain relief.
- Decrease anxiety.
- Experience no complications.

NURSING PROCESS: THE PATIENT WITH INFLAMMATORY BOWEL DISEASE

Assessment

- Onset, duration, and characteristics of abdominal pain.
- Presence of diarrhea, fecal urgency, tenesmus, nausea, anorexia, or weight loss.
- Family history.
- Dietary patterns including alcohol, caffeine, and nicotine use.
- Bowel elimination patterns and characteristics.
- Allergies, especially to lactose.
- Sleep disturbances related to symptoms.

Diagnosis

Nursing Diagnoses

- Diarrhea is related to the inflammatory process.

- Acute pain related to increased peristalsis and inflammation.
- Deficient fluid volume related to anorexia, nausea, and diarrhea.
- Imbalanced nutrition related to dietary restrictions and malabsorption.
- Activity intolerance is related to generalized weakness.
- Anxiety related to impending surgery.
- Ineffective individual coping related to repeated episodes of diarrhea.
- Risk for impaired skin integrity related to malnutrition and diarrhea.
- Risk for ineffective management of therapeutic regimen related to insufficient knowledge.

Collaborative Problems/Potential Complications

- Electrolyte imbalance.
- Cardiac dysrhythmias.
- Gastrointestinal bleeding.
- Perforation of bowel.

Planning and Goals

- Attainment of normal bowel elimination patterns.
- Relief of abdominal pain and cramping.
- Prevention of fluid volume deficit.
- Maintenance of optimal nutrition and weight.
- Avoidance of fatigue.
- Reduction of anxiety.
- Promotion of effective coping.
- Absence of skin breakdown.
- Increased knowledge about the disease process and therapeutic regimen.
- Avoidance of complications.

Nursing Interventions

Maintaining Normal Elimination Patterns

- Provide access to the bathroom.
- Administer antidiarrheal agents.
- Encourage bed rest.

Relieving Pain

- Administer medications as prescribed.
- Provide local application of heat.
- Use diversional activities.
- Prevent fatigue.

Maintaining Fluid Intake

- Monitor intake and output.
- Assess for signs of fluid volume deficit.
- Encourage oral intake.
- Initiate measures to decrease diarrhea.

Maintaining Optimal Nutrition

- Use parenteral nutrition when necessary.
- Provide small, frequent, low-residue feedings.
- Restrict activities to conserve energy.

Promoting Rest

- Recommend intermittent rest periods.
- Encourage activity within limits.
- Perform passive exercises if needed.

Reducing Anxiety

- Tailor information about surgery to the patient's level of understanding.
- Implement stress reduction measures.
- Refer to professional counseling if needed.

Preventing Skin Breakdown

- Examine skin regularly.
- Provide perineal care after bowel movements.
- Use pressure-relieving devices.

Monitoring and Managing Potential Complications

- Monitor electrolyte levels.
- Report dysrhythmias or changes in consciousness.
- Monitor for signs of bowel perforation or obstruction.

Continuing Care

Teaching Patients Self-Care

- Provide information about medications and dietary management.
- Emphasize the importance of medication adherence.
- Recommend use of medication reminders.
- Encourage rest and modification of activities during flare-ups.
- Provide support for coping with the disease.

Evaluation

- Decrease in frequency of diarrheal stools.
- Reduction in pain.
- Maintenance of fluid volume balance.
- Attainment of optimal nutrition.
- Avoidance of fatigue.
- Reduction in anxiety.
- Successful coping with diagnosis.
- Maintenance of skin integrity.
- Understanding of the disease process.
- Absence of complications.

NURSING PROCESS: THE UNCONSCIOUS PATIENT

Assessment

- Evaluate level of consciousness using Glasgow Coma Scale.
- Assess verbal responsiveness, pupil size, equality, and reaction to light.
- Identify spontaneous, purposeful, or nonpurposeful responses.
- Rule out paralysis or stroke.
- Examine respiratory status, reflexes, and body functions systematically.

Diagnosis

Nursing Diagnoses

- Ineffective airway clearance.
- Risk for fluid volume deficit.
- Impaired oral mucous membranes.
- Risk for impaired skin integrity.

- Impaired tissue integrity of cornea.
- Ineffective thermoregulation.
- Impaired urinary elimination.
- Bowel incontinence.
- Disturbed sensory perception.
- Interrupted family processes.

Collaborative Problems/Potential Complications

- Respiratory distress or failure.
- Pneumonia.
- Aspiration.
- Pressure ulcer.
- Deep vein thrombosis.
- Contractures.

Planning and Goals

- Maintenance of a clear airway.
- Protection from injury.
- Attainment of fluid volume balance.
- Achievement of intact oral mucous membranes.
- Maintenance of normal skin integrity.

- Absence of corneal irritation.
- Effective thermoregulation.
- Effective urinary elimination.
- Bowel continence.
- Accurate perception of environmental stimuli.
- Maintenance of intact family or support system.
- Absence of complications.

Nursing Interventions

Maintaining the Airway

- Establish and ensure ventilation.
- Position patients laterally or semiprone.
- Remove secretions and elevate the head of the bed.
- Promote pulmonary hygiene.
- Monitor and maintain the patency of the airway.

Protecting the Patient

- Provide padded side rails and identify potential sources of injury.
- Protect patient's dignity and privacy.
- Act as a patient advocate.

Maintaining Fluid Balance and Managing Nutritional Needs

- Assess hydration status and meet fluid needs.
- Administer IV fluids and blood transfusions cautiously.
- Provide enteral feedings if unable to swallow.
- Monitor intake and output.

Providing Mouth Care

- Inspect and cleanse your mouth regularly.
- Provide oral care for patients with endotracheal tubes or mechanical ventilation.
- Perform oral care interventions to prevent pneumonia.

Maintaining Skin and Joint Integrity

- Turn and reposition regularly.
- Provide passive exercise to prevent contractures.
- Keep joints and legs in proper alignment.
- Use specialty beds to decrease pressure on bony prominences.

Preserving Corneal Integrity

- Cleanse eyes and instill artificial tears.
- Use cold compresses cautiously.
- Avoid contact with cornea and use eye patches cautiously.

Maintaining Body Temperature

- Adjust the environment to promote normal body temperature.
- Treat hyperthermia or hypothermia as prescribed.

Preventing Urinary Retention

- Palpate or scan bladder regularly.

- Insert catheter if signs of urinary retention are present.
- Monitor for skin irritation and breakdown.

Promoting Sensory Stimulation

- Provide sensory stimulation to overcome sensory deprivation.
- Maintain usual day and night patterns of activity and sleep.
- Touch, talk, and involve family members in patient care.

Meeting the Family's Needs

- Reinforce and clarify information about a patient's condition.
- Encourage ventilation of feelings and concerns.
- Support family in decision-making process.

Monitoring and Managing Potential Complications

- Monitor vital signs and respiratory function.

- Assess for adequate red blood cells and initiate chest physiotherapy as needed.
- Perform oral care interventions for patients receiving mechanical ventilation.
- Monitor for skin integrity and implement strategies to prevent pressure ulcers.
- Monitor for signs of deep vein thrombosis and provide appropriate care.

Evaluation

- Clear airway and appropriate breath sounds.
- No injuries.
- Adequate fluid balance and healthy oral mucous membranes.
- Normal skin integrity and absence of corneal irritation.
- Effective thermoregulation and urinary elimination.
- Absence of diarrhea or fecal impaction.
- Appropriate sensory stimulation and coping by family members.
- Absence of other complications.

NURSING PROCESS: THE PATIENT WITH KIDNEY STONES

Assessment

- Evaluate pain and discomfort severity, location, and radiation.
- Assess associated symptoms: nausea, vomiting, diarrhea, abdominal distention.
- Observe signs of urinary tract infection and obstruction.
- Check urine for blood and strain for stones.
- Focus history on predisposing factors for urinary tract stones.
- Assess the patient's knowledge about renal stones and prevention.

Diagnosis

- Nursing Diagnoses: Acute pain, Deficient knowledge.
- Collaborative Problems/Potential Complications: Infection, Obstruction.

Planning and Goals

- Goals: Pain relief, prevention of recurrence, absence of complications.

Nursing Interventions

- Relieving Pain: Administer analgesics, assist with comfort measures, encourage ambulation.
- Monitoring and Managing Complications: Encourage fluid intake, monitor urine output, strain urine, instruct on reporting symptoms.
- Promoting Home- and Community-Based Care: Educate on prevention, fluid intake, follow-up care, and signs of complications after procedures.

Providing Home and Follow-Up Care After ESWL

- Instruct on fluid intake, signs of complications, dietary instructions, and follow-up care.

Continuing Care

- Monitor treatment effectiveness, assess understanding of complications and prevention strategies, ensure awareness of symptoms, and educate on medication actions and side effects.

Evaluation

- Expected Outcomes: Pain relief, increased knowledge, absence of complications.

VEIN DISORDERS

Risk Factors

- History of varicose veins, hypercoagulation, neoplastic disease, etc.
- Obesity, advanced age, oral contraceptive use.

Clinical Manifestations

- Edema, warmth, tenderness, cordlike venous segment.
- Homans' signs, signs of pulmonary embolism.
- Thrombus of superficial veins produces pain, redness, and warmth.

Assessment and Diagnostic Methods

- History, ultrasonography, phlebography.

Prevention

- Identify risk factors, educate patients.

Medical Management

- Pharmacologic Therapy: Heparin, LMWH, oral anticoagulants, thrombolytics.
- Endovascular Management: Thrombectomy, vena cava filter.

Nursing Management

- Assessing and Monitoring Anticoagulant Therapy: Administer heparin cautiously, monitor coagulation tests.
- Monitoring and Managing Potential Complications: Assess for bleeding, monitor platelet counts, provide comfort measures.
- Positioning the Body and Encouraging Exercise: Elevate legs, perform leg exercises, encourage ambulation.
- Teaching Patients Self-Care: Instruct on compression stockings, medication adherence, and monitoring.

GLOSSARY

AIDS (Acquired Immunodeficiency Syndrome)

HIV (Human Immunodeficiency Virus): A retrovirus that attacks the body's immune system, specifically CD4 cells, leading to AIDS if left untreated.

Retrovirus: A type of virus that carries its genetic material in the form of RNA and uses the enzyme reverse transcriptase to convert its RNA into DNA within a host cell.

CD4 (T) cells: White blood cells that play a central role in the body's immune response. HIV infects and destroys CD4 cells, impairing the immune system's ability to fight off infections and diseases.

Primary infection: The initial stage of HIV infection, characterized by flu-like symptoms that occur within 2 to 4 weeks after exposure to the virus.

HIV asymptomatic: The stage of HIV infection where individuals may not experience any symptoms, but the virus is actively replicating and damaging the immune system.

HIV symptomatic: The stage of HIV infection where individuals may experience symptoms such as fever, fatigue, weight loss, and swollen lymph nodes due to the progressive weakening of the immune system.

Opportunistic infections: Infections that occur more frequently or severely in individuals with weakened immune systems, such as those with AIDS.

HAART (Highly Active Antiretroviral Therapy): A combination of antiretroviral drugs used to suppress HIV replication, slow the progression of the disease, and prevent opportunistic infections.

Chemoprophylaxis: The use of medications to prevent the development of infections, particularly opportunistic infections, in individuals with compromised immune systems.

Kaposi's sarcoma: A type of cancer that can develop in people with AIDS, characterized by abnormal growth of blood vessels and purple lesions on the skin or internal organs.

Neurocognitive disorders: Conditions affecting cognitive function, such as memory, attention, and reasoning, often seen in individuals with advanced HIV infection.

Cryptococcal meningitis: An opportunistic infection caused by the fungus Cryptococcus , which affects the membranes surrounding the brain and spinal cord.

Progressive multifocal leukoencephalopathy (PML): A rare and often fatal brain infection caused by the JC virus, typically occurring in individuals with severely weakened immune systems.

Enzyme immunoassay (EIA): A screening test used to detect antibodies to HIV in blood or saliva samples.

Western blot assay: A confirmatory test used to confirm the presence of HIV antibodies in individuals who test positive on an initial screening test.

Viral load test: A blood test used to measure the amount of HIV RNA in the blood, indicating the level of viral replication and effectiveness of treatment.

Saliva test: A rapid HIV test that detects antibodies to HIV in saliva samples, providing results in minutes.

Wasting syndrome (Cachexia): Unintentional weight loss, weakness, and fatigue associated with advanced HIV infection, often accompanied by chronic diarrhea or chronic weakness with fever.

Antidepressant therapy: Treatment involving psychotherapy and pharmacotherapy, including antidepressant medications, to manage symptoms of depression.

Nutrition therapy: A tailored diet aimed at addressing specific nutritional needs and managing symptoms associated with AIDS-related complications, such as diarrhea and weight loss.

Gerontologic considerations: Factors to consider when providing care to elderly patients, including the prevalence and impact of anemia on function and well-being in older adults.

Sickle cell anemia: A severe hemolytic anemia resulting from the inheritance of the sickle hemoglobin (HbS) gene, characterized by abnormal red blood cells that can obstruct blood flow and cause tissue damage.

Assessment: Comprehensive evaluation of the patient's condition, including questioning about precipitating factors, examination of body systems, and monitoring of laboratory values.

Diagnosis: Identification of nursing diagnoses based on assessment findings, which may include acute pain, risk for infection, risk for powerlessness, and deficient knowledge.

Planning: Setting goals for the patient, such as pain relief, decreased incidence of crises, enhanced self-esteem, and absence of complications.

Intervention: Implementation of nursing interventions focused on pain management, infection prevention, coping skills promotion, and patient education.

Monitoring: Regular assessment and observation of the patient's condition, including vital signs, pain level, signs of infection, and laboratory values.

Complications: Potential adverse events that may arise during sickle cell crisis, including hypoxia, infection, dehydration, cerebrovascular accident, anemia, renal failure, heart failure, pulmonary hypertension, impotence, poor compliance, and substance abuse.

Gerontologic Considerations: Specific considerations for elderly patients, such as recognizing common age-related complications like abdominal aortic aneurysms and tailoring care accordingly.

Home- and Community-Based Care: Involving patients and their families in education about disease management, treatment, assessment, and monitoring for complications, along with promoting continuity of care and providing guidelines for seeking urgent care when necessary.

Surgical excision: Removal of tumors or affected tissues through surgical procedures to prevent further growth or metastasis.

Radiation: Treatment using high-energy radiation to target and destroy cancer cells, typically used as adjuvant therapy after surgery or as a primary treatment for inoperable tumors.

Chemotherapy: Administration of drugs to kill cancer cells or prevent their proliferation, often used in combination with other treatments to maximize effectiveness.

Limb-sparing procedures: Surgical techniques aimed at removing cancerous tissues while preserving the functionality of limbs, reducing the need for amputation.

Palliative treatment: Symptom management and supportive care provided to relieve pain and discomfort, improve quality of life, and alleviate suffering, especially for patients with metastatic bone cancer.

Pain management: Implementation of strategies to alleviate pain and discomfort, including administering medications, providing comfort measures, and teaching relaxation techniques.

Patient education: Providing information and instructions to patients and their families regarding their condition, treatment options, self-care practices, and symptom management.

Emotional support: Offering empathy, encouragement, and psychological assistance to patients and their families to help them cope with the challenges of their illness and treatment.

Rehabilitation: Providing assistance and resources to help patients regain functional abilities, mobility, and independence after illness, injury, or surgery.

Multidisciplinary approach: Collaborative effort involving various healthcare professionals from different specialties to provide comprehensive care and address the diverse needs of patients with neoplasms of the musculoskeletal system.

Clinical Manifestations: Identify symptoms like joint pain, fever, rash, and cardiac involvement.

Diagnostic Methods: Conduct throat cultures, assess ASO titers, and perform echocardiograms.

Antibiotic Therapy: Administer antibiotics to eradicate streptococcal infection.

Anti-inflammatory Treatment: Prescribe NSAIDs or corticosteroids to manage inflammation and symptoms.

Symptom Relief: Provide comfort measures for joint pain and fever.

Education: Instruct on antibiotic adherence, importance of follow-up care, and prevention of recurrent infections.

Dietary Guidance: Collaborate with dietitians to develop individualized meal plans tailored to sodium and fluid restrictions.
- Provide education on reading food .

Insidious onset: Gradual or subtle beginning of symptoms over time.

Right lower quadrant abdominal pain: Pain located in the lower right side of the abdomen.

Diarrhea: Frequent and loose bowel movements.

Abdominal tenderness: Pain or discomfort in the abdominal area upon pressure.

Abdominal spasm: Involuntary muscle contractions in the abdomen.

Crampy pains: Sharp and intermittent abdominal pains.

Malnutrition: Lack of proper nutrition due to inadequate intake or absorption of nutrients.

Chronic diarrhea: Persistent and long-lasting diarrhea.

Abscesses: Collection of pus in tissues, often caused by bacterial infection.

Fistulas: Abnormal connections or passageways between organs or tissues.

Fissures: Small tears or cracks in the lining of the anus.

Extraintestinal symptoms: Symptoms affecting areas outside the intestines.

Arthritis: Inflammation of the joints.

Skin lesions: Abnormalities or changes in the skin.

Ocular disorders: Eye-related conditions.

Oral ulcers: Sores or lesions in the mouth.

Barium study: Imaging procedure using barium contrast to visualize the upper gastrointestinal tract.

Endoscopy: Procedure to examine the inside of the digestive tract using a flexible tube with a camera.

Colonoscopy: Examination of the colon and rectum using a flexible tube with a camera.

Biopsies: Removal of tissue samples for microscopic examination.

 examination: Visual examination of the rectum and sigmoid colon.

CT scan: Computed tomography scan, a detailed imaging technique using X-rays to create cross-sectional images.

Stool examination: Analysis of stool samples for abnormalities, such as blood or pathogens.

Blood tests: Laboratory tests to assess various blood parameters, including inflammation markers.

Initiation: Early stage of acute renal failure.

Oliguric: Stage characterized by reduced urine output.

Diuretic: Stage marked by increased urine output.

Recovery: Stage where kidney function begins to improve.

Critical illness: Severe medical condition requiring intensive care.

Lethargy: State of drowsiness or decreased alertness.

Hyperkalemia: Elevated levels of potassium in the blood.

Blood tests: Laboratory tests to assess kidney function and electrolyte levels.

Dialysis: Medical procedure to remove waste and excess fluid from the blood when the kidneys are unable to do so.

Nutritional support: Providing essential nutrients to support overall health during acute illness.

Dear Readers,

Your feedback and support mean the world to us. As authors dedicated to providing valuable resources for nursing students, your input is incredibly valuable. If you've had the chance to preview our book on KDP Amazon, we would be immensely grateful for your thoughts and impressions. Your reviews help us improve and guide future readers towards the resources they need to succeed in their nursing journey. Thank you for taking the time to share your insights with us.

Warm regards,
[Author 1 **Dr. Joshua G. Kaya and Author 2 Dr Brandi J. Gresham**]

www.ingramcontent.com/pod-product-compliance
Lightning Source LLC
Chambersburg PA
CBHW050045230526
45470CB00004B/1415